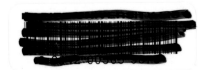

Clinical Geriatric Eyecare

Clinical Geriatric Eyecare

Edited by

Sheree J. Aston, O.D., M.A., Ph.D.
Associate Professor
Pennsylvania College of Optometry
Philadelphia, Pennsylvania

Joseph H. Maino, O.D., F.A.A.O.
Chief, VICTORS Regional Low Vision Center
Department of Veterans Affairs Medical Center
Kansas City, Missouri
Clinical Associate Professor
Department of Ophthalmology
University of Kansas Medical Center

With 5 contributing authors

Butterworth–Heinemann
Boston   London   Oxford   Singapore   Sydney   Toronto   Wellington

Copyright © 1993 by Butterworth–Heinemann

⊋ A member of the Reed Elsevier group

Reed Publishing (USA) Inc. All rights reserved.

Every effort has been made to ensure that the drug dosage schedules within this text are accurate and conform to standards accepted at time of publication. However, as treatment recommendations vary in the light of continuing research and clinical experience, the reader is advised to verify drug dosage schedules herein with information found on product information sheets. This is especially true in cases of new or infrequently used drugs.

Recognizing the importance of preserving what has been written, it is the policy of Butterworth–Heinemann to have the books it publishes printed on acid-free paper, and we exert our best efforts to that end.

Library of Congress Cataloging-in-Publication Data

Clinical geriatric eyecare / edited by Sheree J. Aston, Joseph H. Maino ; with
  5 contributing authors.
      p.   cm.
  Includes bibliographical references and index.
  ISBN 0-7506-9320-7 :
  1. Geriatric ophthalmology. I. Aston, Sheree J. II. Maino, Joseph H.
  [DNLM: 1. Eye Diseases—in old age. 2. Eye Diseases—therapy.
  3. Geriatrics.   WW 620 C641 1993]
RE48.2.A5C55 1993
618.97'77—dc20
DNLM/DLC
for Library of Congress   93-10351
                                            CIP

British Library Cataloguing-in-Publication Data

A catalogue record for this book is available from the British Library.

Butterworth–Heinemann
80 Montvale Avenue
Stoneham, MA 02180

10 9 8 7 6 5 4 3 2 1

Printed in the United States of America

To my parents, Dolly and Jim
and to my staff, Jeanne and Georgia.

Sheree

Time is really the only important currency in life.
Time to frolic with your children.
Time to date your wife.
Time to enjoy the wonders of our world.

Once time is spent there are no refunds.

I need to thank Bunny, David and Christina for allowing me
to spend their time writing this book.

Joseph

Contents

Contributing Authors

Bruce I. Gaynes, O.D.
Private Practice
Chicago, Illinois

Timothy Harkins, O.D.
Staff Optometrist
Department of Veterans Affairs Medical Center
Kansas City, Missouri

Mary Jo Horn, O.D.
Staff Optometrist
Department of Veterans Affairs Medical Center
Fayetteville, Arkansas

Timothy T. McMahon, O.D.
Assistant Professor of Ophthalmology and Visual Sciences
    and Director of Contact Lens Service
University of Illinois at Chicago
College of Medicine
Chicago, Illinois

Rachel Negris, O.D.
Clinical Optometrist
Harvard Community Health Plan
Boston, Massachusetts

Foreword

It is an honor to write a foreword for a textbook. I have always wanted to write one, and in the back of my mind I have always wondered how a person is chosen to write one. Now, I know. In this morning's mail I received a survey from a popular magazine asking me to reply to the following question: Do you think rock and roll is dead? This afternoon I picked up my first pair of bifocals with a teasing note from my own optometrist. It was a quote from Lev Trotsky slipped cleverly into my eyeglasses case. In his *Diary in Exile* (1935), he wrote that "old age is the most unexpected of all things that happen to a man." My wife insisted on putting the note on our refrigerator door for our children to see. So now you see why I now know why Drs. Aston and Maino chose me to write this forward to *Clinical Geriatric Eyecare*. I am nearly qualified.

A number of texts are devoted to the art and science of gerontology. For eyecare providers, they tend to fall into two distinct groups. They are either academic, voluminous, and technically complex, or they are so abbreviated and vague that they offer no real content for clinicians. This is not the case with *Clinical Geriatric Eyecare*, which fills the void eloquently.

In 1990, I was joined by 75 million other "baby boomers" who have entered their presbyopic years. In addition, and during this same year, 31 million Americans were over age 65. By the time I reach 65 over 15% of the population will be just like me. These numbers are staggering.

Doctors Aston and Maino know their subject well, but more importantly they know their readers well. Each of the ten chapters has been carefully selected not only to focus on a subject in gerontology, but also and more importantly to reinforce the overall theme of providing excellence in eyecare for older Americans. Any chapter could stand alone or be read by itself and can additionally serve as a reliable and ready reference for the future. However, it is a mistake to read *Clinical Geriatric Eyecare* in this manner. This text is worthy of one complete read before it is placed among your reference works. It is essential to obtain the broad view of this important subject before settling into its more specific content areas.

The first two chapters written by Dr. Aston set the tone for the text. The remaining eight chapters pay homage to the individual aspects of health and eyecare necessary to provide care for older patients. In particular, the chapters on medications in the elderly, managing older patients with hearing impairments, and addressing elderly patients with cognitive impairments are most welcome and necessary. Geriatric eyecare demands a broad base of clinical knowledge, heightened awareness of aging, and an arsenal of other skills that we rarely think of in the context of caring for older patients. Clearly, Drs. Aston and Maino are cognizant of what we need to know to become better clinicians for our older patients, and they have written this information in a highly readable, concise format. I heartily encourage your initial reading of this text and then your referring to it in your daily practice.

As for my own optometrist, I have forwarded him a thank-you note for my new eyeglasses. I also enclosed a quote written by Sir Walter Raleigh the night before his death in 1618, which was subsequently found in his Bible.

> Even such is Time, which takes in trust
> Our youth, our joys, and all we have,
> And pays us but with age and dust;
> Who in the dark and silent grave,
> When we have wandered all our ways,
> Shuts up the story of our days:
> And from which earth, and grave, and dust,
> The Lord shall raise me up, I trust.

John W. Potter, OD

Preface

Only recently have the nation's schools and colleges of optometry provided formal education in geriatric optometry. Most of today's practicing optometrists have received little or no didactic information on assessing and managing the eye and vision problems of the older adult. Yet, knowledge of how to care for the needs of elderly patients is crucial for proper optometric care.

Clinical Geriatric Eyecare was written to provide practical information to help care for the rapidly increasing number of geriatric patients seen in practice. This comprehensive but focused text guides you through basic and advanced clinical procedures to help simplify your professional life while improving the quality of patient care.

The authors have provided useful information based on personal clinical experience and in-depth research. This "how-to" text is a guide to caring for the geriatric patient and is intended for all practice settings from the private one-doctor office through the multidoctor, multispecialty institutional clinic. Specifically, this book provides information to (1) help you effectively market your practice to the geriatric patient, (2) improve your office setting to enhance your care, (3) improve the quality of care, (4) work with such institutions as nursing homes and specialty clinics, and (5) care for older patients with multiple impairments.

The book is organized to help you quickly find the information you need. A brief introduction acquaints you with basic demographics and statistics. Next we walk you through office and communications design to make care for the older patient "user friendly." Chapters 3 through 5 deal directly with patient care and offer vital general information necessary for geriatric eyecare. Finally, chapters 6 through 10 discuss such specialty areas as geriatric low vision rehabilitation and contact lenses and important information on how to help the older patient with multiple impairments.

In summary, this clinically oriented guide is meant to be used by all doctors who care for one of this country's greatest treasures—our senior citizens.

S.J.A.
J.H.M.

1

The Elderly Population

Sheree J. Aston

The elderly population continues to increase in size faster than any other American age group. This demographic phenomena is often referred to as the "graying of America." Older adults in the United States are and will continue to be a major influence on this country in general and health care and the practice of optometry in particular (Aston, 1990).

The number of geriatric individuals in the United States has increased dramatically in this century. The percentage of Americans aged 65 and older has tripled, from 4.1% in 1900 to 12% in 1985. This striking growth in our nation's elderly population is due primarily to decreased infant mortality, preventive health care measures, advanced life-saving technology, and improved clinical medicine (Fowles, 1986).

In 1990, the population of persons aged 65 years or older was reported to total 31.2 million. This group is so large and diverse it has been categorized recently into three age groups: young-old (65–74), middle-old (75–84), and old-old (85 years and older). Typically, these groups differ in their social, economic, and health characteristics. The oldest of the old are by far the largest consumers of social, health, and vision care services (Davis and Kirkland, 1986; U.S. Senate, 1988; AOA, 1990).

FUTURE POPULATION GROWTH

By the year 2000, the elderly population is expected to total 34.9 million, representing 13% of the entire U.S. population. By 2030, more than one in five individuals will be senior citizens (AARP, 1991), and between 1990 and 2040, the elderly population will more than double. More astonishing is the growth in the number of the "oldest of the old," those aged 85 years and older, which will more than double by the year 2010 and triple before 2030 (U.S. Senate, 1983).

LIFE EXPECTANCY

The average life expectancy for Americans has grown tremendously during the twentieth century. In 1900, Americans lived an average of 47 years, whereas a child born in 1989 has a life expectancy of 75.2 years. The major reason for

1

this increase is the reduction in infant mortality and improvement in health status of older adults. An elderly person who reached his or her 65th birthday in 1989 will most likely live an additional 15 to 20 years (AARP, 1991).

ECONOMIC STATUS

Households headed by an elderly person reported an average income of $25,105 in 1990. Furthermore, 10% of these households had an income of $10,000 or less and 40% had an income of $30,000 or more. In 1988, the leading sources of income for older Americans in descending order were social security (39%), asset revenue (25%), personal earnings (17%), and retirement pensions (17%) (AARP, 1991).

Contrary to common perceptions, the elderly as a group are wealthier, not poorer, than the general population. The median net worth of elderly households was $73,500, compared with the 1988 national average of $35,800. The net worth of households was less than $10,000 for 17% and was above $250,000 for 14% of the elderly group (AARP, 1991).

HEALTH AND HEALTH CARE

The majority of the elderly are healthy, functional, and live in the community. In fact, only 5% of adults 65 and older reside in institutional settings, although most older adults (85%) do have at least one chronic health problem and more than half have two or more conditions (Brody, 1986). In 1989, the ten leading health problems of noninstitutionalized elderly were arthritis (48%), high blood pressure (38%), hearing impairment (29%), heart disease (28%), cataracts (16%), orthopedic impairment (16%), sinusitis (15%), diabetes (9%), vision impairment (8%), and varicose veins (8%) (AARP, 1991).

In 1987, the elderly constituted 12% of the population yet consumed 36% of personal health care services in the United States. The largest expenditures were for hospitals (42%), followed by physicians' fees (20%) and long-term care (20%) (AARP, 1991).

The number of noninstitutionalized elderly who need assistance with activities of daily living (eating, dressing, shopping, walking, and so on) increases with age. Fourteen percent of persons aged 65 to 74 need assistance. A much higher proportion of individuals 85 years and older (48%) need help in these activities (U.S. Senate, 1988).

VISION CARE AND THE ELDERLY

Historically, the elderly population has been considered to include individuals aged 65 years and older based on the standard eligibility criteria for social security and medicare. Practically, optometrists and other health care providers are interested in the number of *older* adults (55 years and older). In 1990, the U.S. Census estimated the 55-and-older group to be approximately 53 million persons, more than one in five of the living individuals in the United States. This trend toward aging of the population will continue through the year 2030. There will be 61 million older (55 +) Americans by the year 2000 and 75 million by the year 2010—more than one of every four persons in the United States! (AOA, 1990).

The vision care needs of these adults are immense. The incidence and prevalence of normal and abnormal visual changes increases with age. The vast majority of older Americans will require optometric services for the following reasons: almost all will be presbyopic, 65% to 70% will be astigmatic, 60% will be hyperopic, 20% will be myopic, most will have spots and floaters, and a large number will experience dry eye. Furthermore, more than 15% will have senile cataracts, almost 9% will have age-related maculopathy, 3% will have diabetic retinopathy, and 2% will have glaucoma (AOA, 1990).

The combination of optometric parity in medicare and the enormous growth of the elderly population will have a formidable effect on the optometric practices. The flow of older adults into optometric practices will change the patient base of most providers. Therefore, optometrists will need to have special knowledge, skills, and techniques to deal effectively with this population in their offices, the community, and institutional settings.

REFERENCES

American Association of Retired Persons and the Administration on Aging. A Profile of Older Americans: 1991. Washington, American Association of Retired Persons, 1991.

American Optometric Association. Who are older Americans? AOA News 1990; p. 7.

Aston SJ. The graying of America: Optometric considerations. Introduction. Optometry and Vision Science 1990; 67(5):313–314.

Davis LJ, Kirkland M. The Role of Occupational Therapy with the Elderly. Rockville, The American Occupational Therapy Association, 1986.

Fowles D. Profile of Older Americans. Washington, American Association of Retired Persons and the Administration on Aging, 1986.

U.S. Senate. A Report of the Special Committee on Developments in Aging: 1982. Washington, U.S. Government Printing Office, 1983.

U.S. Senate, the American Association of Retired Persons, Federal Council on Aging, and the U.S. Administration on Aging. Aging America: Trends and Projections. Washington, U.S. Department of Health and Human Services, 1988.

2

Overall Practice and Patient Management Strategies

Sheree J. Aston

Some older adults will experience illnesses that may require eye care in the home or in an institutional setting; however, the vast majority will receive optometric services in a private office or clinic. This chapter will provide the information necessary to build and maintain the geriatric practice. Strategies are described on how to participate in the aging network, communicate effectively, modify office practices, create a comfortable and safe environment, and provide services in a conducive atmosphere.

Demographics demonstrate that the older patient will have a profound effect on the practice of optometry. In their zenith years, optometrists graduating in the 1990s will have the elderly constituting two thirds to three quarters of their practices. This population is significant not only because of its size, but also because of its wealth. The 55- to 64- and 65- to 74-year-old groups have the highest assets and net worth of all adult age groups (U.S. Bureau of the Census, 1986).

Networking is a useful tool for the optometrist to use to both *build* and *maintain* a successful geriatric practice. It involves interacting with a variety of formal and informal resources in order to provide or assess geriatric knowledge or services. Planned correctly, it is also extremely valuable in "getting and keeping" the older patient. Knowing how to locate the elderly individual, redesign an office, provide a comprehensive service, and act as a resource broker are necessary for a successful geriatric optometric practice.

ATTRACTING SENIOR PATIENTS

Building a geriatric practice involves locating the elderly in the vicinity of the practice, making contacts, increasing visibility of eye care, providing senior discounting, formal/informal education, pooling resources, and modifying staffing patterns.

Finding seniors involve several steps. First, identify specific areas around the optometric practice where older persons reside. This includes certain neighborhoods, retirement villages, or life-care communities. A local library or college library will usually have copies of 1990 U.S. Census. This will give details of the age groups for particular areas in the vicinity of the practice. It will give information on exact census tracts as well as block units. The second way of locating new seniors is by making contact with the local welcome wagon and real estate brokers or by monitoring new housing developments such as life-care communities and retirement villages. Practitioners should concentrate on geriatric populations within 15 to 20 minutes of their practice. The literature reports that older consumers will not drive more than 20 minutes for their services. Finally, each "senior rich" area should be targeted for optometric marketing materials (Scipione, 1989).

Making Contacts

Making contact begins with learning about the geriatric centers and services available in the local community. Request literature from state and community organizations on aging to determine what services, programs, and organizations are in the immediate locale. Send a letter that provides information on the senior-geared optometric office to these nearby geriatric organizations and centers. Follow up with appointments with these organizations to educate their staff about vision and aging and services provided by the private practice. Personal contacts with these organizations will be strongly related to future referrals, linkages and overall networking.

Increasing the Visibility of Eye Care

Optometrists can increase the visibility of their practices and at the same time provide valuable community services by performing public educational activities including free vision screenings, distribution of informative materials, and professional presentations at local senior organizations and centers. Suggested topics for the materials and seminars are normal vision and aging changes, functional implications of normal changes, importance of routine eye care, how to identify vision problems, low vision and aging, and aging and driving. It is important to provide education to the staff at these organizations on such additional topics as signs and symptoms of vision problems, environmental design for visually impaired adults, resources for visually impaired adults, travel skills for visually impaired adults, networking within the eye care field, and improving the visual functioning of the older adult.

Vision Screenings

Vision screenings are an excellent sources of referrals for optometric practices. Settings to be considered include churches and synagogues; civic groups (Lions Clubs, Rotary Clubs, and Kiwanis); American Association of Retired Persons (AARP) chapter meetings; Gray Panther chapter meetings; senior centers; day care centers; senior citizen clubs; and life-care communities. Screenings are best conducted mid-morning, well before lunch time. A large room that can be darkened is best for the location. An on-site staff member of the center or organization should make the preliminary arrangements for the room and appointments. Use the optometric staff to assist in the screening activity to maximize the doctor's time. A written questionnaire on the health history should be completed prior to the screening.

Typical screenings include ocular and systemic health history, visual acuity at distance and near, pupil evaluation, tonometry, and direct ophthalmoscopy. An exit interview should be conducted with the patient to discuss normal and abnormal findings. A written recommendation for an evaluation or referral must be provided for each patient, the sponsoring organization, and the practitioner's office file. Additional vision testing can be provided at the optometrist's office (Aston and Mancil, 1989).

Pooling Resources

Another way to reach the elderly is by pooling local resources. Optometrists should network within their community with other health care providers. Find out which dentists, physical therapists, physicians, podiatrists, and pharmacologists in the local community seek to devote a greater portion of their services to the older adult. Volunteer to be part of a team to make public education presentations or conduct in-service seminars, distribute educational materials, and provide comprehensive screenings to age-related organizations. Interoffice referrals can be achieved easily by this health service network. Educational materials on optometric services can be placed in the "team" offices to generate additional geriatric patients.

Other Strategies

An optometrist educated in gerontology is most attractive to the older person. Geriatric courses including certificate programs are usually available at local colleges or community colleges. Informal education about older adults can be gained by reading periodicals such as *Money Magazine, Psychology Today, Forbes,* the *Wall Street Journal,* the *AARP Journal* and professional publications from the following geriatric organizations: American Society on Aging, the Gerontological Society of America, and the National Council on Aging. Employing a staff member aged 55 or older also sends a strong, positive message to the elderly individual. Older people will be more comfortable in setting appointments, completing forms, and providing a history when interacting with someone of their own age.

Another mechanism to build and maintain a senior practice is through personal referrals. A new patient who has a positive experience at an optometric practice will tell friends and family about a geriatric-friendly service. It is appropriate to thank the referring patient with a card or other gesture of appreciation.

A final suggestion to attract seniors to the optometric office practice is to offer a discount on the eye examination, frames, and/or lenses at the first visit.

Practitioners should also consider dedicating a slow day as "senior day" for the practice. This type of information can be included on the bottom of any educational materials or newsletters distributed to the geriatric organizations and individuals.

COMMUNICATION

Understanding and interacting with the older person is essential to any geriatric practice. Many optometrists find elderly people difficult to deal with in their private practices, but problems are often based upon misunderstandings stemming from poor communication. Effective communication is one of the most critical elements in proper patient management. It forms the foundation for a successful doctor-patient relationship. According to Sullivan and Meyers (1976) a major factor in patient satisfaction is based on the doctor's skill in patient communication, not on time spent with the patient.

Communication begins with the first contact between the prospective older patient and the optometric office. The initial telephone inquiry sets the tone for the relationship. Staff members must be trained to speak respectfully, using formal titles. Speech should be slow, clear, and slightly louder (without shouting) in order to be understood by the mildly hearing-impaired person. When the geriatric patient enters the office, the receptionist should quickly and warmly greet the person, assisting with a person's coat or seating if necessary. All staff should be observant of the person's mood, facial expressions, speech, reaction to the office environment, and ability to move around. This information will be helpful to the doctor in providing care. Time in the reception area can be spent completing preliminary information forms, which will assist in the examination. This also sends the message that the elderly individual's time is considered valuable. Proper information exchange is vital throughout the entire examination process.

Other useful tips for communication with older individuals follow:

- Directly face the individual when speaking.
- Use simple phrases and short sentences (without being condescending).
- Speak in a lower pitched voice.
- Address the patient as "Mr." or "Mrs." (unless otherwise instructed).
- Express interest in personal safety and comfort and offer assistance whenever needed.

The History

History-taking is a unique opportunity to build rapport and trust between the doctor and the patient. The use of questions that will elicit only a yes or no answer often will not cover all pertinent information needed for the examination. Open-ended questions are best for the interview phase of the evaluation. Because of normal age-related delayed responses, additional time must be allowed for answering questions. At first, patients should be allowed to converse freely. This action will demonstrate genuine feelings of interest and caring; however, the doctor must control the interview, and if necessary, impose limits on the conversation. Patients who appear to ramble may actually be concealing a fear that they are not expressing regarding an eye problem. Make sure to discover the real reason for the visit by asking, "What brought you to the office today?" (Barresi, 1985).

Communication skills needed to deal effectively with an older person are different than with other individuals. Verbal and written exchanges with an older adult are often affected by age-related problems such as hearing loss, reduced vision, poor memory, delayed response time, fatigue, physical difficulties, or confusional states such as senile dementia of the Alzheimer type (Dancer, 1985). Doctor-patient communication can be enhanced by following the strategies suggested by Dancer (1985):

- Repeat instructions.
- Present the information in a slower fashion.
- Allow the person adequate time to respond.
- Have a period of conversation before testing to reduce anxiety.
- Use techniques of positive reinforcement, encouragement, and slight touch.
- Write instructions in large, bold type.

Patient Education

Patient education begins early in the reception area with informative material and should be woven throughout the entire examination. The older patient must be an active participant in the assessment process. Both normal *and* abnormal findings need to be related to the patient. Compliance will undoubtedly be increased in the case of an educated patient. Patient education also comes into play when the need for following a treatment regimen is reinforced. The patient who understands *how* and *why* a certain medication is needed is more likely to follow prescribed treatment strategies.

Messages on the importance of routine eye care and age-related vision problems can be transmitted to geriatric patients through a variety of brochures. The American Optometric Association has a selection of pamphlets on vision and aging, presbyopia, and driving tips and the elderly, as well as on specific age-related eye diseases. Another suggestion is to develop original patient educational materials. Educational flyers can cover topical areas such as color, contrast, and lighting in the home, the latest treatment for various eye diseases, advances in cataract surgery, and information on new ophthalmic products. It would be worthwhile to survey patients on other topics of interest. Practitioners should consider creating newsletters that can be sent to geriatric patients on these same subjects. Use the following guidelines for development of patient educational materials:

- Use short sentences with simple wording.
- Use large print with good contrast to paper.
- Describe topics in simple rather than technical terms.
- Increase white space by using double or triple spacing with wide margins.
- Keep language at fourth grade or lower to increase comprehension.
- Avoid the use of blue, violet, or green colored paper or printed word.
- Do not use reflective or glossy paper for materials.

Elderly patients should understand that many of the vision problems they are experiencing are normal to the aging process. Problems with the glare and night driving, the perception of certain colors, and focusing at near can all be explained as the result of normal changes. The educated patient will adjust more easily to these types of changes.

Optometrists must be careful about informing a patient of a diagnosis, such as cataract. Many people become alarmed when they hear the words *cataract, glaucoma,* or *presbyopia.* Diagnoses must be simply and completely explained to patients in terms they can easily understand. The older patient should be educated and treated as an adult and *not* a child. Proper patient education will increase overall patient satisfaction levels.

OFFICE DESIGN

The environment of optometric practices must be modified to meet the needs of the geriatric persons. These considerations include easy outside access and interior design that focuses on comfort and safety.

Access and Passageways

Older patients have a preference for practices that are easy to locate and have adequate parking close to the office entry. Access from the parking area to the door of the practice should be accomplished with a minimum of effort. The entrance to the practice preferably will have no or few steps and a ramp for easy accessibility of wheelchairs. Entry to the building and/or suite should be through a doorway that is easily negotiated by a person in a wheelchair. The door should have a handle at convenient height that pulls rather than turns to open. A path of adequate width from the entrance to the reception area and to the examination room is needed (Anstice, 1986). Typically, interior designers plan office space by accepted standards, but the elderly often need more space because of physical limitations or to accommodate their assistive devices. Five feet across is required to permit two-way passage of wheelchairs or a patient assisted by another individual. In planning reception and examination rooms, the rule of thumb is to increase regular standards by a factor of one fourth to one third (Jordan, 1984).

Arrangement of furniture should also allow for easy movement of persons with assistive devices. At least a portion of the reception counter should be waist level for the wheelchair-bound patients. The reception area, hallways, and examination rooms should be uncluttered to allow for maneuvering of persons with walkers and wheelchairs. The entire office, including the restrooms, should be accessible to the handicapped. Restrooms should be located as close to the examination area as possible.

Interior Design

Office decor should be designed with the elements of color, contrast, and lighting in mind. Good use of color and contrast is a must in printed office materials (Mancil, 1990). Older persons surveyed have indicated a preference for bright, rather than pale or pastel, colors. Do not use green, blue, and violet; they are less distinguished by the aging eye (Mancil, 1990). Because of natural age-related changes in the ocular media, reflective surfaces such as chrome, mirror or glass should also be avoided. Nonglare, nonslip floor coverings are best used whenever possible to prevent falls.

Adequate contrast in wall to floor interfaces, steps, and any signage is necessary. Do not choose counters, furniture, and walls to match the color of the carpets and other interfacing areas. This is dangerous for persons with impaired vision. It is vital that adjacent surfaces such as doors, door frames, and walls have good color contrast. Exposed pipes should also have distinctive colors that can be discriminated by older individuals.

Proper lighting in the entire office area is especially critical to individuals with normal and abnormal visual, hearing, and physical limitations. Incandescent or natural lighting is recommended to reduce glare and improve visual acuity. This is especially helpful in the reception or waiting areas where patients normally complete pre-examination forms or read leisure and educational materials.

Vinyl wall coverings are preferable to paint because they are decorative, durable, and more easily maintained. Older individuals are more likely to use the wall for support, and vinyl surfaces are much easier to keep clean. Wall coverings, upholstered furniture, draperies, and carpeting should be used to reduce background noise, which is disturbing to older individuals with the normal age-related hearing deficits. Acoustical ceiling tile is also another way to lower sound levels.

Comfort and safety are important considerations in selecting furniture for the office. Soft comfortable sofas and chairs are often difficult to get into and even harder to get out of. Chairs should be 17 inches above the floor with a width of 20 inches between the arms. The depth should not exceed 16 inches. The backs of couches, if used, should be at least 21 inches above the floor and have full back support.

Chair and couch arms are essential and should extend a few inches beyond the front of the furniture. It is difficult for an older person to reach a coffee table from a seated or standing position, so instead use side tables approximately 29 inches high (Jordan, 1984). Follow Jordan's (1984) suggested guidelines when designing the optometric office or clinic:

- Encourage independent functioning.
- Compensate for visual, auditory, and physical changes.
- Provide a safe, comfortable environment.
- Increase accessibility of service.

A thoughtful and informed office design can greatly improve the comfort level of an older person and can be achieved without decreasing the independence of the elderly.

OFFICE PRACTICES

Successful care of older patients involves modification of pre-examination protocols, examination techniques, and the overall management plan. It is recommended that staff be trained on the normal and abnormal changes with aging and how this effects everyday life. Age-related sensory loss, especially vision, should be covered in detail.

Staff can also serve as resources to older patients if they become familiar with special agencies and services available in the local community (see the networking section of this chapter). Consider educating office employees in communication techniques and other skills necessary to work effectively with all patients, especially older ones. Of course, employment of an older person is an asset to any office that deals with elderly patients.

Pre-examination Protocols

Older persons must be treated with special care and respect. A variety of magazines, journals, and books of interest to the older patient should be available in the waiting room, along with periodicals and magazines in large print for both older and visually impaired persons. Provide informative brochures and pamphlets, on a variety of pertinent vision and age-related subjects for the reception area. The time spent in the reception area can also be used to complete pre-examination questionnaires. Collect data on all medications (including over-the-counter drugs) as well as a complete family history and personal health history. In the case of a confused patient, a family member or friend may be asked to gather missing details. If additional history is needed from a significant other, the preferred setting is in the private office without the patient present.

Scheduling is a major component in setting the stage for a successful doctor-patient interaction. The appointment should be arranged for a time convenient to the older patient, in the morning if possible to avoid problems with fatigue. The doctor is also freshest at this time of the day. Evening and Saturday hours are also much appreciated by the older person who is dependent upon a working friend or family member for transportation to the office. An appointment should allow enough time for a longer evaluation. It is not uncommon to require a second visit to finish the examination of an older patient. In that case the full fee should be charged for the first appointment with the second being free of charge (Cole and McConnaha, 1986).

The Examination

During the examination, keep the patient informed about the nature and purpose of various tests and procedures. It is important to take the time to let patients know of normal as well as abnormal findings. In order to reduce a patient's anxiety during a refraction, indicate the lack of "right" or "wrong" answers.

The patient's perception of competence is often based on the *quality* of time spent in the evaluation without interruption. Fifteen minutes of intense time, without distraction by staff telephones or background noise, will result in increased patient satisfaction, reduce a patient's fear about the examination, and enhance the perception of the doctor's clinical ability (Cole and McConnaha, 1986).

Do not leave the examination room without telling the older patient. It is unwise to leave the elderly patient in a raised chair with the lights off. In the doctor's absence, make sure that patients are aware of the location of the restroom. This is necessary considering that incontinence is more common among the aged (Cole and McConnaha, 1986).

Patient Compliance and Management

The management plan may be ineffective because of poor patient compliance. Common reasons for noncompliance by older adults include poor understanding or misunderstanding of the ocular condition, importance of treatment regimen, or directions for drug usage. The existence of a hearing loss or confusional state will also decrease patient compliance. Noncompliance often can be handled by improving communication. Techniques for improving communication and therefore compliance are easy to incorporate into everyday practice.

Any therapeutic intervention should be thoroughly explained to the patient. Consider the following scenario: Mr. Greene, age 70, is diagnosed with glaucoma, yet is experiencing no symptoms. It is crucial that Mr. Greene understand and expect possible side effects from the medications. The long-term consequences of untreated glaucoma must be clearly stated to the patient. Mr. Greene should be asked to repeat his understanding of his condition, treatment plan, and instructions for self-medication. Dr. Jones can further emphasize the management plan by written communication in clear and large print. It is not uncommon for a patient to misunderstand due to sensory problems or pure age-related forgetfulness. In the case of a confused patient, the diagnosis and the treatment regimen should also be discussed with family members or significant others.

It can benefit patients to demonstrate their ability to instill eye drops before they leave the office. It will increase their confidence and ability to self-medicate. The decision regarding assistance by family or friend could be made at that time by the doctor (Mancil, 1990).

NETWORKING: ACTING AS A
RESOURCE BROKER

The other side of networking is to serve patients by becoming knowledgeable about the formal aging system. Doctors of Optometry can be a vital link to services and programs needed by the older adult because often optometrists are the initial or only contact between older patients and health care and social fields. Optometric practitioners, as health care primary providers, have an opportunity to serve as referral agents and coordinators of multidisciplinary care. All health care providers need to form associations with the aging network in order to prevent illness, promote wellness, and improve the functioning and the overall quality of life for their older patients.

The *aging network* is a formal outgrowth of the Older Americans Act, enacted in 1965, which was developed to improve the quality of life for older persons. It was designed to provide services and information in income, health, housing, employment, retirement, law, and recreation. The Administration on Aging is the federal unit responsible for overall direction of grant programs and services authorized through the Older Americans Act (Titles II and III). There are ten regional offices as well as units of aging in the fifty states and several commonwealths. The state units administer rather than deliver any direct services or programs; they provide guidance and funding through local Area Agencies on Aging (AAA).

There are more than 660 AAAs in the United States. They can be located in the blue pages of the telephone book. AAAs may deliver services themselves or contract to local providers. AAAs develop, coordinate, and provide programs and services for persons over the age of 60. They also act as advocates for the elderly and furnish information and referrals services as needed. AAAs receive funding and guidance from the state units along with a combination of other local, state, and federal funds.

All AAAs do not have identical services and programs. They have different offerings based on their own program plans. Examples of the variety of services include telephone assurance, homemaker services, transportation, information and referral, friendly visitor program, home health care, legal services, senior centers, senior citizens club, daycare centers, respite care centers, and home-delivered meals. It is not uncommon for vision services to be provided through a contract with a local optometrist or ophthalmologist. This is within the realm of services provided to the elderly if AAA administrators are aware that this is a common problem to be addressed.

Another resource in networking are professional organizations devoted to the elderly population. Contact the state and local chapters of the following national groups to form linkages to attract and build the geriatric optometric practice:

Geriatric Associations. The National Council on Aging, Gerontological Society of America, the National Association Area Agencies on Aging,

American College of Healthcare Administrators, and American Society on Aging.

Health Organizations. The American Dental Association, the American Medical Association, the American Nurses Association, the American Occupational Therapy Association, the American Physical Therapy Association, the American Society of Allied Health Professionals, the American Society of Consultant Pharmacists, and the National Association of Social Workers.

Volunteer Programs. The American Association for Retired Persons (AARP), the Community Service Employment Program, and Retired Senior Volunteer Program.

It is necessary for the optometrist to network both in the aging and health field to deliver quality, comprehensive care to the older patient. Successful networking will enable the optometric practitioner to build and maintain a solid geriatric practice with satisfied older patients.

REFERENCES

Anstice J. Vision care in the home and institutional setting. *In* Rosenbloom R, Morgan M (eds): Vision and Aging: General and Clinical Perspective. New York, Fairchild Publications, 1986.

Aston S, Mancil G. Community health issues in optometric gerontology. *In* Aston S, DeSylvia D, Mancil G (eds):Optometric Gerontology: A Resource Manual. Rockville, Association of Schools and Colleges of Optometry, 1989.

Barresi B. Optometric assessment of the aged—general principles. *In* Bleimann R (*ed*): Workbook on Optometric Gerontology. St. Louis, American Optometric Association, 1985.

Cole K, McConnaha D. Understanding and interacting with older patient. American Optometric Association Dec 1986;57(12):82–87.

Dancer J. General considerations in the management of older persons with communication disorders. *In* Jacobs-Condit L (ed):Gerontology and Communications Disorders. Rockville, American Speech-Language Hearing Association, 1985.

Jordan J. The challenge: Designing buildings for older Americans. Aging Dec 1983–Jan 1984;99–102.

Mancil G. Serving the needs of older patients through private practice settings. Optometry and Vision Science May 1990;67(5):315–318.

Scipione P. Capturing and keeping the senior patients. Optom Manage Nov 1989:42–48.

Sullivan WA, Meyers R: How to see more patients in less time. Optometric Management May 1976;12(5):147–149.

U.S. Bureau of the Census. Household Wealth and Asset Ownership:1984. Current Population Reports 1986, July series, no. 7, p. 70.

3

The Elderly and Medications

Bruce I. Gaynes
Sheree J. Aston

The elderly often experience multiple chronic illnesses and require numerous medications, often with complicated dosing schedules. Consider the following characteristics of the elderly regarding medications:

- 71% use prescription medications (DeSylvia et al., 1989; Pagliaro and Pagliaro, 1983)
- 54% use over-the-counter drugs (DeSylvia et al., 1989; Pagliaro and Pagliaro, 1983)
- 25% take four or more prescription medications (DeSylvia et al., 1989; Pagliaro and Pagliaro, 1983)
- 25% of all prescribed medications are used by the elderly (DeSylvia et al., 1989; Pagliaro and Pagliaro, 1983)
- 50% of the elderly's health care budget is spent on prescription and over-the-counter drugs (DeSylvia et al., 1989)

The result of such reliance on medication has problems in that the elderly are uniquely susceptible to adverse drug reactions and drug toxicity. As the use of medications by the elderly increases, the frequency of drug-induced illnesses and toxicity will proportionately accelerate. Changes in physiology that occur with age and their relationship to drug pharmacokinetics and dynamics alter anticipated drug action. Unfortunately, economic and social changes are frequent problems encountered by the elderly, which can also complicate effective drug therapy.

What physiologic changes occur as we age that would adversely affect drug action and how do these changes relate to effective use of medications in the elderly? The answers to these questions lie in understanding basic pharmacologic principles of drug action.

PHYSIOLOGY, PHARMACOKINETICS, AND THE ELDERLY

The size of dose administered is an important factor in the magnitude of response obtained; however, these relationships fail to tell us what proportion of the total dose actually is responsible for the final drug action. Moreover, it fails to tell us what intermediate factors have occurred that lead to the final drug concentration and the desired effect. There are basically three processes responsible for final drug concentration at the receptor site: drug absorption, distribution, and elimination. These processes occur as a function of time and may be influenced by factors such as biotransformation, drug binding, and the chemical nature of the drug in question. The study of a drug's rate of absorption, distribution, and elimination is collectively termed *pharmacokinetics*. The establishment of a latent period, time to peak effect, duration of action, and biologic half-life all are influenced by pharmacokinetics (Gwilt, 1990).

Alterations in pharmacokinetics in elderly patients is associated with physiologic aspects of aging, particularly in the liver, kidney, and gastrointestinal (GI) system. The majority of drug absorption occurs in the GI system, particularly in the stomach and intestine. In the stomach, typical aging changes seen after age 50 that may be responsible for decreased drug absorption include atrophy and thinning of mucosa and accelerated and sustained cell turnover, which lead to decreased secretion of mucous important for protective and absorptive functions. Elevation of gastric pH in the aging stomach may alter ionization and solubility of various drugs. Decreased blood flow due to congestive heart failure, hypoxia, and hypovolemia lead to ischemia and arterial occlusion, which may also diminish drug absorption (Lamy, 1989).

The elderly show decreases in gastric emptying, which may be a consequence of lack of ambulation, gastric ulcers, diabetes mellitus, myocardial infarction, or stress (Bhanthumnavin and Schuster, 1977). Although a decrease in gastric emptying may be thought of as increasing drug absorption, total drug absorption is actually decreased because of the inability of the drug to reach the high absorptive capacity of the intestines, which also may undergo degenerative age changes similar to those as seen in the stomach.

Once a drug reaches the blood compartment it is distributed to its target organ. The rate at which the drug penetrates tissues and body fluids to reach the receptor site depends on several factors: (1) rate of blood flow (perfusion), (2) extent and amount of plasma protein drug binding, (3) regional differences in pH, (4) transport mechanisms available, (5) permeability characteristic, (6) tissue mass, and (7) volume of distribution (Vd). Drug distribution may be altered in the elderly due to changes in the body composition. The elderly tend to have less body water and more total body fat, which reduces the proportion of actual lean body mass per unit body weight (Forbes, 1976). The elimination half-life varies with the ratio Vd/drug clearance. Drugs that are distributed mainly in body water or lean body mass (e.g., antimicrobial agents, digoxin, lithium) would be expected to have a lower Vd versus lipid soluble drugs and may attain higher serum concentrations than anticipated. Lipid soluble drugs such as neuroleptic agents have an increased Vd in the aged with a subsequent increase in half-life.

Inconsistencies in Vd make plasma half-lives difficult to predict and less useful as a measure of drug elimination in the aged.

Many drugs are carried to their target tissues by plasma proteins, which have been noted to decrease with age (Rafsky and Brill, 1952). Protein binding plays a role in regulating free drug available for drug-receptor interaction and drug elimination. As the amount of free plasma protein decreases, the levels of free drug increase, which may act to exert a stronger pharmacologic response.

Drug metabolism and elimination are also responsible for influencing drug concentration at the receptor site. When absorbed from the GI tract, a drug must pass through the portal circulation before reaching the systemic blood compartment. This hepatic "first-pass effect" is responsible for a large percentage of drug metabolism and in some cases, drug elimination. The liver, which is considered to be the primary organ of chemical detoxification, plays a large role in drug clearance. This is achieved through a series of enzymatic reactions termed *biotransformation*. It is of interest that the same type of biotransformation enzyme systems found in the liver are also found in the eye, particularly the iris and ciliary body, where they likely function in similar manner in the metabolic clearance of topically applied ophthalmic agents.

The effects of aging on hepatic drug metabolism are difficult to predict. The physical condition of the patient is of most importance in evaluating hepatic clearance. Clinically, it is important to note that normal liver serum chemistry analysis, however informative, does not directly reflect the status of hepatic metabolic integrity.

Drug elimination, the final component considered in the development of a clinically acceptable drug regimen, is primarily the function of the kidney and is a result of complex renal physiology. The aging kidney undergoes a number of changes in morphology and physiology, including a decrease in the number of functioning nephrons, a decrease in glomerular filtration and renal blood flow, and a decrease in creatinine clearance (Dunhill and Halley, 1973). Histologic changes, perhaps related to chronic disease states, include fibrous or hyaline transformation of the glomeruli, distention and atrophy of the tubules, and changes in the interstitial connective tissue and vascular supply (Andrew and Pruett, 1987). It is noteworthy that animal studies by Davies et al. (1989) found few morphologic changes in aged mice and implicated chronic disease conditions in most of the qualitative changes found in the aged human kidney. Whatever the cause, decrease in renal function can affect pharmacokinetics of drugs and their metabolites excreted by the kidney. A decrease in renal function results in delayed drug clearance and prolonged half-life, contributing to drug toxicity.

DRUG INTERACTIONS

The normal physiologic and acquired pathophysiologic changes that occur in the elderly not only complicates single drug administration but potentiates drug-drug interactions and adverse drug effects as well. Elderly patients often visit several physicians for illnesses that require a variety of medications. This ultimately leads to polypharmacy and potentiates drug-drug interactions (Lamy,

1986). Although pharmacists are well trained in the detection of potential drug-drug interactions, the use of mail-order drug services and "price comparison" shopping often leads the patient to several outlets for drug purchases. In addition, the elderly patient often over-utilizes nonprescription medications in an attempt to self-medicate and perhaps circumvent the necessity for a costly but needed visit to a doctor's office or clinic. These over-the-counter medications are notorious for interfering with the action of important prescription drugs and delaying accurate diagnoses. It should be noted, however, that not all drug interaction is bad, nor is the concomitant use of several drugs in one patient always harmful. For example, the delay in excretion of penicillin produced by probenecid may prolong the antimicrobial effect of the former. The use of several drugs in the treatment of glaucoma is common and an effective means of controlling the disease.

Knowledge of the pharmacologic actions of each specific drug aids in the selection of agents that result in synergism or potentiation rather than antagonism. For example, agents such as anticoagulants, oral hypoglycemics, antiarrhythmics, and digitalis-type drugs have narrow windows of therapeutic effectiveness; therefore, relatively small changes in their plasma concentration produced by drug interactions can have disastrous effects. Drugs such as the benzodiazepines, however, may not pose such a serious threat due to their wider margin of safety. In the treatment of open angle glaucoma, concomitant use of topical and systemic beta blockers may result in serious depression of cardiac function and exacerbation of respiratory distress.

ADVERSE DRUG REACTIONS

There is a certain danger when any drug, however beneficial, is prescribed. Drug-drug interactions and unexpected, idiosyncratic adverse drug actions are a frequent cause of iatrogenic illness. This is particularly true in the elderly who, for reasons just discussed, are more susceptible to side effects and unwanted actions of drugs. Studies have shown the incidence of adverse drug reactions increases with age and the number and frequency of drug-dose exposures. About 30,000 deaths and 1.5 million hospital admissions per year result from adverse actions of drugs. Moreover, one in five hospitalized geriatric patients suffers ailments directly related to their prescribed medication, whereas one in nineteen patients over age 50 is admitted to the hospital due to drug-induced illness (Peterson and Thomas, 1979).

The practitioner must establish the value of a particular drug for therapeutic use through consideration of a risk-benefit ratio, without which no value can legitimately be given to using any medication. Although the value of most drug therapy is usually apparent, uncertainty may occur in cases of unorthodox or experimental drug therapy or with drugs that have narrow margins of safety. Consideration of variables such as the margin of safety, potency, concentration, and toxicity of the drug in question, as well as the physical condition of the patient, must be linked. The nature of the toxicity should also be a consideration in view of the condition treated. For example, aplastic anemia found with the use of ophthalmic chloramphenicol may be considerably more serious than a bacterial conjunctivitis. Drug choice obviously requires serious thought of all variables. Familiarity of potential drug-induced side effects is important for early recognition and avoidance of iatrogenic illness. Once again the relationship between pathophysiology and functional physiologic changes plays an important role in predicting drug toxicity. Seriousness of potential toxicity is an important consideration in selecting drugs. Drugs prescribed for chronic use must be evaluated for the possibility of future as well as immediate adverse actions.

Individuals who are most at risk for adverse drug reactions are 75 years of age and older, female, small in stature, taking multiple medications, suffering from kidney dysfunction, and using high-risk drugs. Signs of adverse reactions include confusion, weakness, lethargy, ataxia, forgetfulness, tremor, constipation, and anorexia. Some examples of potential drug-induced side effects resulting from commonly prescribed drugs are presented in Table 3-1.

USE AND MISUSE OF DRUGS
Successful Drug Therapy

One of the most important considerations in the success of any therapeutic agent is patient recognition of the need for care, coupled with prompt access to the appropriate health care practitioner. Elderly patients often delay entering the health care system because of lack of accessibility, economics, or apathy. Self-medication also delays appropriate diagnosis, which can hamper the correct medical treatment. Once the patient makes contact with the health care practitioner, an examination is performed and a diagnosis is made. The outcome of any drug regimen is dependent on the appropriate diagnosis in conjunction with an acceptable therapeutic plan. Blanket or "shotgun" approaches of drug therapy often results in inappropriate medication use, iatrogenic drug illness, or hampering of the correct diagnosis.

Consideration of other concurrent illnesses and drug use must be given before prescribing in order to avoid unwanted and unnecessary drug-drug and drug-induced adverse reactions. In addition, some drugs may interact with intrinsic disease processes, leading to an exacerbation or initiation of medical problems, which only further complicates drug therapy. Information regarding any type of allergy to drugs, food, and so on is crucial to the therapeutic decision. The elderly often exhibit anxiety in visiting the doctor, and care should be given to relieve tension, making sure the patient understands his or her current condition, possible need for further tests, and necessary medications. All too often prescriptions are written for conditions the patient has no knowledge of or vaguely understands, which leads to poor compliance. Communicate in a friendly and open manner and in a such a way that the patient understands the need for medication and when and how to take it. Often a pharmacist reemphasizes pertinent points of the particular drug(s) prescribed and makes certain the patient understands the proper use of the medication.

Table 3-1   Adverse Drug Reactions

Type of Drug	Common Adverse Reactions
Analgesics	
Anti-inflammatory agents	Gastric irritation
	Chronic blood loss
Narcotic	Constipation
Antimicrobiais	
Aminoglycosides	Renal failure
	Hearing loss
Levodopa	Nausea
	Delirium
Anticholinergics	Dry mouth
	Constipation
	Urinary retention
	Delirium
Cardiovascular	
Antiarrythmics	Diarrhea (quinidine)
	Urinary retention (disopyramide)
Anticoagulants	Bleeding complications
Antihypertensives	Sedation and/or other changes in mental function
	Hypotension
Calcium channel blockers	Decreased myocardial contractility
Diuretics	Dehydration
	Hyponatremia
	Hypokalemia
	Incontinence
Digoxin	Arrhythmias
Hypoglycemic agents	
Insulin	Hypoglycemia
Oral agents	Hyponatremia (chlorpropamide)
Psychotropic agents	
Lithium	Weakness
	Tremor
	Nausea
	Delirium
Antipsychotics	Sedation
	Hypotension
	Extrapyramidal movement disorders
Sedative and hypnotic agents	Excessive sedation
	Delirium
	Gait disturbances
Other drugs	
Aminophylline	Gastric irritation
	Tachyarrhythmias
Cimetidine	Mental status changes
Terbutaline	Tremor

Reprinted with permission from Kane et al. Essentials of Clinical Geriatrics. New York, McGraw Hill Information Services, copyright © 1989.

Noncompliance

In most ambulatory clinical settings, once the patient receives the prescription and leaves the doctor's office the responsibility of obtaining the medication and using it appropriately rests with the patient. Compliance is a particular problem with the elderly because many aged patients face obstacles in obtaining and using medication that are often complex and compounded by social, economic, psychological, and physical conditions. Problems such as macular degeneration, stroke, and senile dementia all contribute to problems in patient compliance because of physical and intellectual limitations. These physical problems must be dealt with in day-to-day situations and may be compounded by social and economic factors.

When prescribing medication it is important that the practitioner consider such factors before dismissing the patient. Other important factors include easy to open bottles and legibly written instructions. Review drug use by the patient at every follow-up visit and, if possible, observe the patient's use of the drug, particularly eyedrops, which are often difficult to instill. Patients with poor vision may benefit from bright, color-coded containers or specialized containers to regiment dose scheduling. Home health aides or visiting nurses can also help to dispense medication correctly. Make certain the patient realizes that these types of services may be available if needed. Compliance will be improved by unhurried communication and familiarity with all problems facing the patient's proper use of medications.

OCULAR PHARMACOLOGY

Due to anatomic and pathologic ocular changes seen with aging, elderly patients often require more scrutiny to determine the effectiveness of a prescribed medication and observe any possible adverse actions. For example, changes in eyelid structure such as involutional entropion and ectropion may alter duration of drug contact. The cornea becomes less sensitive with age, and patients may not "feel" a drop of medication placed on the eye. Keratitis sicca, common in the geriatric population, may enhance drug absorption due to punctate corneal erosions. A myriad of adverse actions can complicate drug therapy, particularly in the elderly, and may lead to therapeutic failure. The optometrist should be familiar with medications commonly used in geriatric ophthalmic practice and their actions, both desired and adverse.

Autonomic Agents—Cholinergic Drugs

Cholinergic drugs have long been utilized as ocular hypotensive agents in the treatment of various glaucomas. They are fairly safe drugs from the standpoint of systemic toxicity and rarely cause serious side effects (apart from the indirect agents); however, adverse reactions may develop in susceptible individuals. Systemic adverse reactions and contraindications to the use of cholinergic drugs both direct and indirect include hyperthyroidism, coronary insufficiency, and peptic ulcer. Cholinergic agents are noted for their bronchoconstrictor effects and may precipitate an asthma attack in predisposed individuals. Cholinergic agonists may increase bronchial secretions, which may also exacerbate an asthmatic condition. Toxicity may produce salivation and lacrimation as well as nausea and vomiting. Doses of 10 to 15 mg of pilocarpine may produce marked diaphoresis, nausea, vomiting, and weakness. Assuming 20 drops/mL, a 2% pilocarpine solution contains 1 mg/drop. It may be readily seen that in acute angle closure glaucoma, for example, in which pilocarpine instillation occurs frequently, toxicity must be carefully assessed. Examples of commonly used cholinergics include pilocarpine, carbachol, and the indirect acting parasympathomimetics, physostigmine, demecarium, and isofluorophosphate.

Parasympatholytics

The prototype drug for parasympatholytics agents is atropine. Adverse reactions vary in severity and are associated with the potency and dose of the particular agent questioned. Systemic effects from topical ophthalmic application can occur and include difficulty in urination, constipation, cardiac arrhythmias, and central nervous system toxicity, which is more prevalent in children and infants and includes disorientation, hallucinations, and delirium. Facial flushing and fever may be noted, along with extreme dryness of the mouth.

Ophthalmic effects include cycloplegia and mydriasis. A rise in intraocular pressure may be seen in patients who have glaucoma, both open and narrow angle. This is particularly important in narrow angle glaucoma in which use of these agents may enhance bunching of the iris root into the angle, further enhancing mechanical angle closure. In addition, atropine may increase aqueous outflow resistance in eyes with open angle glaucoma.

Sympathomimetics

Systemic absorption of topically applied ocular sympathomimetics such as epinephrine may result in heart palpitation, hypertension, and cardiac arrhythmia. In addition, headache, tremor, anxiety, and nervousness may be noted. Topical ocular application of catecholamines has been found to induce or exacerbate macular edema following cataract extraction and is contraindicated postoperatively after cataract extraction. Pigment abnormalities in the form of dot-like brown-black adrenochrome deposits, resembling foreign bodies, may form on the lower palpebral conjunctiva. They often become encapsulated by squamous epithelium and cause no symptoms; however, pigment deposits on the upper tarsal conjunctiva may become large and cause corneal irritation. Epinephrine therapy may cause mydriasis, and caution should be taken when employing epinephrine for the treatment of glaucoma in patients with shallow anterior chambers.

Dipivefrin is a congener of epinephrine, a prodrug converted to epinephrine by metabolic enzymes within the eye. Dipivefrin is available as a 0.1% solution for the treatment of open angle glaucoma. The same precautions and adverse actions must be considered as for epinephrine. Phenylephrine is a synthetic noncatecholamine alpha adrenergic agonist with little beta effect. It is a strong vasoconstrictor and is used as a topical ophthalmic decongestant in concentrations from 0.025 to 0.1% It also is used as a mydriatic agent at 2.5 and 10% concentrations. Significant hypertensive crises may occur upon systemic absorption of topical ocular application, particularly of the 10% viscous solution. Systemic toxicity includes marked reflex bradycardia secondary to the rise in diastolic blood pressure; however, little cardiac stimulation occurs. Particular care should be used when phenylephrine is administered to elderly patients with pre-existing cardiovascular problems and severe arteriosclerotic conditions. As with all adrenergic drugs, concurrent use with monoamine oxidase (MOA) inhibitors should be avoided for a period of up to 21 days following MOA therapy because exaggerated adrenergic response may result. Guanethidine and reserpine may also exacerbate hypertensive crises with concurrent adrenergic administration. Baseline blood pressure measurements may be helpful before instillation of phenylephrine in elderly hypertensive patients. In addition, most commercial 2.5% phenylephrine solutions are preserved with a bisulfite compound that presents additional allergic risk in sensitive individuals, particularly asthmatic patients.

Apraclonidine (paraminoclonidine) is a relatively new alpha adrenergic agonist that has been released as an agent to control or prevent intraocular pressure elevation postsurgically. The drug has been found to be effective in controlling the elevation of intraocular pressure following such procedures as argon laser trabeculoplasty, argon laser iridotomy, or Nd:YAG posterior capsulotomy (Robins, 1991). It may also induce mydriasis but is not used clinically for this purpose. It has little direct action on the heart. It is similar to the drug clonidine, which acts centrally to activate alpha$_2$ receptors, resulting in reduced peripheral sympathetic tone and a consequent decrease in blood pressure (Hoskins and Kass, 1989).

Sympatholytics

Systemic adverse actions upon topical ophthalmic application of the beta blockers can result in significant morbidity if careless prescribing habits occur. Adverse actions include bradycardia, hypotension, congestive heart failure, syncope, exacerbation of bronchial asthma, psychic disorientation, and confusion. Up to 10% of patients receiving timolol may suffer from one or more of these iatrogenic conditions (Van Buskirk, 1980). Care should be used in prescribing these agents in elderly patients with pre-existing cardiac or respiratory disease. As a precaution before starting ophthalmic beta blocker therapy, obtain baseline blood pressure, pulse, and electrocardiograph (ECG) in elderly patients, along with a medical consultation, if deemed necessary.

Timolol is, perhaps, the most widely used nonselective beta receptor antagonist available for topical use in the treatment of open angle glaucoma. Levobunolol is also a nonselective sympatholytic used in the treatment of open angle glaucoma with similar cardiovascular effects (Geyer et al, 1988).

Betaxolol is available as a cardioselective agent in the treatment of open angle glaucoma and has been found to have less adverse effects on respiration (Schoene et al., 1984; Buckley et al., 1990). Clinically, the drug displays variable results as far as preventing respiratory depression.

Carbonic Anhydrase Inhibitors

Many side effects of carbonic anhydrase inhibitors are related to renal function. Carbonic anhydrase inhibition may result in an alkaline urine and metabolic acidosis. Hypokalemia in the elderly may lead to cardiac arrhythmia, particularly in those patients receiving digitalis medications. Carbonic anhydrase inhibitors also appear to cause serious hematologic problems including aplastic anemia, leukopenia, pancytopenia, agranulocytosis, and thrombocytopenia. Most problems with blood dyscrasia develop within 6 months of therapy. Questioning the patient about bruising, excessive bleeding, and frequency of infections may lead the practitioner to suspect the development of hematologic problems. Frequent blood tests, particularly in the first 2 or 3 months, while reassuring, may not prevent a hematologic crisis, which is usually idiosyncratic, dose-independent, and unpredictable. A hematocrit, platelet count, and white blood cell count may be run every 2 months for the first 6 months as a precaution (Zimran and Beutler, 1987). In addition, carbonic anhydrase inhibitors should be used with caution in patients known to have sickle cell disease, because drug-induced exacerbation of the condition has been noted. Nephrolithiasis may also occur as a result of calcium deposition in an alkaline urine lacking citrate (Kass et al., 1981; Lichter et al., 1978; Maren, 1967). Acidifying the urine and increasing urine output may protect against nephrolithiasis formation.

Dichlorphenamide and ethoxzolamide are additional carbonic anhydrase inhibitors that may be used as an alternative to acetazolamide (Lichter, 1981). The various agents differ in potency but not efficacy: They all produce the same ocular hypotensive effect with varying doses. The variations in potency are related to differences in lipid solubility and drug-protein binding. Ethoxzolamide is the most potent of carbonic anhydrase inhibitors; however, it is limited in activity due to high protein binding. Methazolamide penetrates more easily into ocular tissue as well as into the central nervous system (CNS). Sedation, fatigue, and drowsiness may be more apparent with this agent. Methazolamide is not, however, taken up by the renal tubules as is acetazolamide; thus the former compound is better tolerated in diabetic patients with concurrent renal disease.

Corticosteroids

Side effects of glucocorticoids can be serious, particularly with systemic use, and include one or more of the following: congestive heart failure, diabetes mellitus, gastric ulceration, osteoporosis, fluid retention, hypokalemia, psychosis, and depression (Hogan et al., 1955). Suppression of the hypothalamic-pituitary-adrenal cortex feedback system is found in long-term therapy, necessitating tapering of the steroid when the medication is discontinued. This also prevents rebound inflammation. Ocular side effects of systemic therapy include cataracts, open angle glaucoma, exaggeration of herpes simplex, increased susceptibility to cytomegalovirus (CMV) retinitis, and in some cases, exophthalmos, papilledema, and ptosis. Topical corticosteroid therapy is not without significant risks and include such problems as decreased corneal wound healing, inhibition of corneal endothelial regeneration, enhancement of herpetic and fungal keratitis, enhancement and exaggeration of bacterial keratitis, open angle glaucoma (more common with topical versus systemic use), and cataracts (Havener, 1983). Steroid-induced glaucoma is, however, reversible in most cases following discontinuation of the corticosteroid agent (Armaly, 1963).

Nonsteroidal anti-inflammatory agents—Flurbiprofen

The flurbiprofen types of nonsteroidal anti-inflammatory agents are effective inhibitors of the cycloxygenase, which is used in the biosynthesis of prostaglandins. In the eye, prostaglandins have been implicated in mediating postoperative miosis and inflammation due to vasodilatin, increased vascular permeability, leukocytosis, and breakdown of the blood-aqueous barrier (Flower et al., 1986). Increased intraocular pressure has also been associated with prostaglandin release (Podos et al., 1973). Although the potential anti-inflammatory benefits of cycloxygenase inhibition are evident, the drug currently is approved only for the prevention of postoperative miosis. The usefulness of flurbiprofen as a topical ocular anti-inflammatory agent has not yet been fully determined.

Antivirals

In the eye, the primary use of antivirals is for infections of the DNA viruses, particularly herpes simplex and to some extent varicella zoster, vaccinia, and CMV. Antivirals work by inhibiting one step in viral replication and are often nonselective in action; however, increased data on how viruses replicate have led to the recent development of more selective and less toxic agents such as trifluridine. Herpes simplex keratoconjunctivitis often responds well to antiviral therapy, but herpes zoster keratoconjunctivitis usually responds to topical steroids, with various topical antivirals being ineffective. Oral acyclovir may, however, be beneficial. Ganciclovir and foscarnet are recently developed agents effective in CMV retinitis. Idoxuridine and vidarabine are two additional agents available in the treatment of herpes simplex keratitis.

Antimicrobials

Aminoglycosides

All aminoglycosides are bacteriocidal and act by inhibiting bacterial protein synthesis. Aminoglycosides apparently have high affinity for renal cortical tissue, which ultimately results in reversible renal insufficiency. Advancing age has been suggested as a risk factor in the development of aminoglycoside-induced renal insufficiency due to an overall physiologic reduction of renal function and concurrent renal disease (Webster et al., 1970; Schentag et al., 1978). Ototoxicity may be cochlear and/or vestibular and may be manifested by vertigo, hearing loss, tinnitus, and unsteady gait. Cochlear toxicity is often irreversible. Topical ophthalmic application of aminoglycosides rarely results in toxicity; however, between 6% to 8% of patients receiving topical neomycin develop a severe hypersensitivity reaction that is cross reactive with other aminoglycosides (Sande and Mandell, 1985). Transient burning upon instillation has been reported; corneal toxicity manifested by a diffuse punctate keratitis has been observed.

Erythromycin

Erythromycin has a spectrum similar to penicillin and is often employed as an alternative to penicillin in allergic patients. *Haemophilus influenzae, Streptococcus, Staphylococcus* and *Mycoplasma* organisms are particularly sensitive; however, resistant *Staphylococcus* organisms frequently may be encountered. It is effective against chlamydia conjunctivitis.

Tetracycline

Tetracycline and its congeners are employed topically as well as systemically in ophthalmic practice for the treatment of chlamydial keratoconjunctivitis and acne rosacea blepharitis and keratoconjunctivitis. GI irritation after oral administration is common with these agents.

Sulfonamides

Sulfonamides are structural analogues of *p*-aminobenzoic acid (PABA), which is necessary for cell growth, and are competitive inhibitors of PABA uptake by the cell. Therefore, since purulent discharge contains high amounts of PABA, they are not indicated in a suppurative bacterial infection. They are broad spectrum agents effective against gram-positive and some gram-negative organisms, as well as *Chlamydia* and *Toxoplasma gondii* organisms. The sulfonamides are antagonistic to gentamicin in the treatment of pseudomonas and they should not be used concurrently in the treatment of pseudomonal conjunctivitis (Burger et al., 1973).

Bacitracin and the Polymixins

Bacitracin is a polypeptide antibiotic produced by *Bacillus subtilis*. It is not inactivated by penicillinase and develops less resistance than penicillin. Corneal penetration is poor. It is unstable in solution and is often used in a combination topical ointment. The polymixins comprise a group of polypeptide antibiotics; two are in commercial use, polymyxin B and polymyxin E (colistin). They are bacteriocidal and work by interfering with cell membrane phospholipid leading to an incompetent bacterial cell wall. Their spectrum is limited to gram-negative bacteria, including *Pseudomonas aeruginosa*.

Fluoroquinolones

Fluoroquinolones make up a recently developed class of ophthalmic antimicrobial agents includes ciprofloxacin and norfloxacin. They are broad spectrum agents effective against the staphylococci, *Hemophilus influenzae, Neisseria, Pseudomonas aeruginosa,* as well as gram-negative bacilli. They have limited effect against the chlamydiae. They are bacteriocidal, interfering with the synthesis of bacterial DNA.

PRINCIPLES OF PRESCRIBING FOR GERIATRIC PATIENTS

Once the practitioner has completed an examination and arrived at a diagnosis, a plan is compiled to help the patient resolve or alleviate his or her particular medical condition(s). More often than not, the plan includes use of prescription drugs that must be taken at various intervals, sometimes on an indefinite basis. The use of medications, particularly in elderly patients, is not without pitfalls. Many drug-related illnesses in the elderly occur due to lack of understanding of the expected changes in drug pharmacokinetics and dynamics of various medications and how they may be further altered by various pathologic conditions. Individual analysis of such functions as drug absorption, plasma protein binding, metabolism, and renal excretion should augment the decision to use specific drug therapy and dosage. In addition, certain drugs used by the elderly may be more apt to cause adverse effects due to their inherent chemical and physiologic properties. Ocular side effects of medications must be considered (Table 3-2).

In general, guidelines for prescribing systemic as well as topical ophthalmic medication in elderly patients include

1. Taking a complete medical and drug history, including known allergies and current prescription medication and over-the-counter drug use (Appendix 3-1).
2. Titrating doses gradually if possible.
3. Individualizing medication, dosage form, and dose and keeping the medication regimen as simple as possible.
4. Paying special attention to individual disabilities, which may interfere with compliance, such as poor vision or impaired intellect. Tamper-resistant containers present a potential problem to an elderly patient.
5. Making certain the patient understands the drug regimen, possible adverse reactions and side effects, and what they are to do if a problem develops. Repeating and writing instructions down are helpful, as is having the patient acknowledge that he or she understands what the medicine is for and what the particular drug regimen is.
6. Making use of relatives, friends, visiting nurses, and pharmacists to help ensure compliance.
7. Using the patient-doctor relationship to the advantage of the practitioner as well as the patient by establishing and keeping open communications

Table 3-2 Ocular Side Effects of Systemic Medications

Drug	Ocular Side Effects
Antiarthritics	
Corticosteroids	Cataract
	Glaucoma
	Impaired corneal wound healing
	Increased risk of viral, fungal, and bacterial infections
Antidepressants	
Lithium	Loss of central acuity
Tricyclic	Ocular muscle imbalances
	Visual hallucinations
Antiepileptics	
Barbiturates	Sluggish pupillary response
	Miosis
	Transient nystagmus
Dilantin	Nystagmus
	Conjunctivitis
	Ptosis
Antihistamines	
	Mydriasis
	Impaired accommodation
	Rarely, angle closure glaucoma
Antipsychotics	
Chlorpromazine	Pigmentation on anterior lens capsule and back of cornea
	Rarely, keratoconjunctivitis.
Thorazine	Pigmentary retinopathy without bull's eye pattern
Cardiac medications	
Digitalis	Color illusions
	Impaired visual acuity
	Flickering vision
Quinidine	Decreased visual field
	Mild decrease in intraocular pressure
Antihypertensive agents	
Chlorothiazide	Xanthopsia
	Acute myopia
Hydralazine	Lid edema
	Lacrimation
	Rarely, decreased visual acuity
Nonsteroidal anti-inflamatory agents	
Ibuprofen	Reduced central acuity
	Optic neuritis
	Diplopia
Indomethacin	Corneal deposits
Salicylic acid	Stevens-Johnson syndrome
	Severe keratitis
	Optic neuritis

Adapted with permission from Brady KD and Ellis PP. Ocular pharmacology. *In* Kwitko ML and Weinstock FJ (eds); Geriatric Ophthalmology. Orlando, Grune and Stratton, 1985.

and by encouraging questions in an unhurried relaxed manner. The elderly sometimes require more patience and often react negatively to a rushed practitioner who lacks time to adequately explain exactly what their condition is and how various medications may help them.

In general, the elderly are more sensitive to the actions of drugs. Alterations in drug metabolism, end-organ response, plasma proteins, and renal clearance all play a role in promoting hypersensitivity. The care of the elderly requires thorough understanding of the many physiologic changes due to aging and how these changes may alter drug response in a particular individual. Chronic disease often exerts various pathophysiologic changes in morphology and function in all tissues and may be indistinguishable or confused with normal physiologic aging changes. Nevertheless, the final endpoint is the same: altered drug disposition. The various homeostatic alterations observed in the elderly may also greatly affect drug use and toxicity. Aging is a complex progressive process involving all organ systems; the elderly are not simply "old" young persons. Individual assessment of each patient's own need and particular problems will decrease drug toxicity, enhance compliance, and allow medications to act as safe and effective tools in prolonging and improving the lives of the elderly.

Acknowledgment

Dr. Gaynes would like to thank his wife, Sara, for her support and invaluable help in the preparation of this chapter.

REFERENCES

Andrew W, Pruett D. Senile changes in the kidneys of Wistar Institute rats. Am J Anat 1987;100:51–79.

Bhanthumnavin K, Schuster M. Aging and gastrointestinal function. *In* Finch C, Hayflick L (eds): Handbook of the Biology of Aging. New York, Van Norstrand Reinhold, 1977, p 209.

Buckley MM, Goa KL, Clissold SP. Ocular betaxolol. Drugs 1990;40:75–90.

Burger LM, Sanford JP, Zweighaft BA. The effect of sulfonamides on the anti-Pseudomonas activity of gentamicin in vitro. Am J Ophthalmol 1973;75:314–318.

Davies J, Fotheringham AP, Faragher BE. Age-associated changes in the kidney of the laboratory mouse. Age Ageing 1989;18:127–133.

DeSylvia DA, Logan SG, Vanderveen RP, Klug ED. Pharmacology/chemical dependency. *In* Aston SJ, Mancil GL, DeSylvia DA (eds): Optometric Gerontology. A Resource Manual for Educators. Rockville, Association of Schools and Colleges of Optometry, 1989.

Dunhill MS, Halley W. Some observations of the quantitative anatomy of the kidney. Journal of Pathology. 1973;110:113–121.

Flower RJ, Moncada S, Van JR. Analgesic-antipyretics and anti-inflammatory agents: Drugs employed in the treatment of gout. *In* Gilman AG, Goodman LS, Rall TW, Murad F (eds): Goodman and Gilman's The Pharmacologic Basis of Therapeutics, 7th ed. New York, Macmillan Publishing, 1985, pp 675–676.

Forbes GB. The adult decline in lean body mass. Hum Biol 1976;48:161–173.

Geyer O, Lazar M, Novack GD, et al. Levobunolol compared with timolol: A four year study. Brit J Ophthalmol 1988;72:892–896.

Gwilt PR. Pharmacokinetics. *In* Craig CR, Stitzel RE (eds): Modern Pharmacology, 3rd ed. Boston, Little Brown, 1990, p 68.

Goldberg I, Ashburn FS, Palmberg PF, et al. Timolol and epinephrine, a clinical study of ocular interaction. Arch Ophthalmol 1980;98:484–486.

Havener WH. Ocular Pharmacology, 5 ed. St. Louis, CV Mosby, 1983, pp 142–147.

Hogan M, Thygeson P, KiMura S. Uses and abuses of adrenal steroids and corticotropin. Arch Ophthalmol 1955;53:165–176.

Hoskins HD, Kass MA. Becker-Shaffers's Diagnosis and Therapy of the Glaucomas, 6th ed. St. Louis, C.V. Mosby, 1989, p. 446.

Kass MA, Kolker AE, Gordon M, Goldberg I. Acetazolamide and urolithiasis. Ophthalmology 1981;88:261–265.

Lamy PP. Elder Care News, Vol 5, pp 26–31. Baltimore, University of Maryland, School of Pharmacy, 1989.

Lamy PP. The elderly and drug interactions. J Am Geriatr Soc 1986;34:586–592.

Lichter PR. Reducing side effects of carbonic anhydrase inhibitors. Ophthalmology 1981;88:266–269.

Lichter PR, Newman LP, Wheller NC, Beall OV. Patient tolerance to carbonic anhydrase. Am J Ophthalmol 1978;85:495–502.

Maren TH. Carbonic anhydrase: Chemistry, physiology, and inhibition. Physiol Rev 1967;47:595–781.

Pagliaro LA. Pagliaro AM. Pharmacologic Aspects of Aging. St. Louis, C.V. Mosby, 1983.

Podos SM, Becker B, Kass MA. Prostaglandin synthesis, inhibition and intraocular pressure. Investigative Ophthalmology 1973;12:426–433.

Petersen DM, Thomas CW. Acute drug reactions among the elderly. *In* Petersen DM, Thomas CW (eds): Drugs and the Elderly, Social and Pharmaceutical Issues. Springfield IL, Charles C. Thomas, 1979, pp 41–50.

Rafsky HA, Brill AA, Stern KG, et al. Electrophoretic studies on the serum of "normal" aged individuals. Am J Med Sci 1952;224:522–528.

Robins AL. Argon laser trabeculoplasty medical therapy to prevent the intraocular pressure rise associated with argon laser trabeculoplasty. Ophthalmic Surg 1991;22:31–37.

Sande MA, Mandell GL. Antimicrobial agents—aminoglycosides. *In* Gilman AG, Goodman LS, Rall TW, Murad F. (eds): Goodman and Gilman's The Pharmacologic Basis of Therapeutics, 7th ed. New York, Macmillan Publishing, 1985, p 1165.

Schentag JJ, Cumbo TJ, Jusko WJ, Plaut ME. Gentamicin tissue accumulation and nephrotoxic reactions. JAMA 1978;240:2067–2069.

Schoene RB, Abuan T, Ward RL, Beasley CH. Effects of topical betaxolol, timolol, and placebo on pulmonary function in asthmatic bronchitis. Am J Ophthalmol 1984;97:86–92.

Van Buskirk EM. Adverse reactions form timolol administration. Ophthalmology 1980;87:447–450.

Webster JC, McGee TM, Carroll R, et al. Ototoxicity of gentamicin. Transactions of the American Academy of Ophthalmology and Otolaryngology 1970;74:1155–1165.

Zimran A, Beutler E. Can the risk of acetazolamide-induced aplastic anemia be decreased by periodic monitoring of blood cell counts. Am J Ophthalmol 1987; 104:654–657.

Interview Guide for Comprehensive Medication Assessment of Elderly Clients

INTERVIEW QUESTION	GUIDES AND RATIONALE
Part I	
1-5 What medications are you taking now?	1-5 A. Have client or family member collect together all medications and bring to you.
	B. Check instructions on label with orders on chart. Check date obtained and expiration dates. Check for multiple prescribing physicians and multiple pharmacies. For any discrepancies or problems noted, probe further for possible reasons.
6. Can you tell me what this medication is supposed to do for your condition?	6. To assess client's knowledge and understanding about the purpose of the prescribed medication and client's need for information.
7. Do you think this medication is working for you?	7. To assess client's beliefs about the efficacy of the prescribed medication.
8. Do you have any concerns about taking this medication?	8. To assess client's concerns about the costs/risks related to the prescribed medications.
	A. High cost of medications
	B. Fear of drug dependence
	C. Adverse or side affects/drug interactions
	D. Ability to obtain (e.g., difficulty getting to pharmacy, lack of transportation)

INTERVIEW QUESTION

GUIDES AND RATIONALE

    E. Interference with lifestyle (e.g., eating habits, religious beliefs, sleep patterns)

    F. Other (specify)

For questions 9-13, probe for specific reasons if discrepancies are noted between prescribed instructions and client's practices.

9. How many times during the day do you take this medication?

9. To assess if the client is taking the medication according to the prescribed practices.

10. When do you take this medication? At what hours or times of the day?

10. To assess if the client is taking the medication at the proper times.

11. How much of the medication do you take?

11. To assess if the client is taking the prescribed amount (dose) of the medication.

12. How are you taking this medication?

12. To assess if the client is taking the medication by the proper route, especially for creams, liquids, and topicals.

13. Are there any medications that you take only as necessary or periodically?

13. To assess if the client is taking PRN medications appropriately and for the proper reasons.

14. Are there any special instructions or precautions you follow in taking this medication?

14. To assess client's comprehension of and adherence to special instructions for self-administration of medications (e.g., don't drive, take only with food).

Part II

15. What other medications/drugs/substances are you taking other than the prescription medications we've been discussing?

15. To assess client use of:
    A. Over-the-counter drugs
    B. Alcohol
    C. Vitamins/nutritional supplements
    D. Other

16. Do you have any of the following difficulties that interfere with you taking your medications:
Opening containers?

16. To assess for functional and sensory impairments that may cause barriers to self-administration of medications.

For suspected deficits, ask client to:
Open container

INTERVIEW QUESTION

Breaking tablets?
Giving eye drops?
Handling syringes?
Reading labels?
Distinguishing colors of pills?

17. Many people have some difficulty in remembering to take their medications. Are there times when you have difficulty remembering to take your medications? Or are there times when you just don't want to remember to take your medications?

18. Do you have some methods (tricks) you use to help you plan or remember to take your medications? Describe what happened the last time you forgot to take your medication. What do you do when you forget to take a dose? Is there anyone here in your home (e.g., spouse) or someone close by who can encourage you or help you to remember to take your medication?

19. Are there any medications that you have stopped taking altogether?

GUIDES AND RATIONALE

Read label to you
Distinguish colors

17. To assess for cognitive/memory or psychological problems (e.g., depression) which may interfere with remembering to take medications.

18. To assess for family/lifestyle or social problems which may interfere with self-administration of medications.

19. To assess for premature medication discontinuation by the client.

Possible reasons:
A. Absence of symptom or symptom improvement
B. Medication fails to improve or relieve symptom
C. High cost of medication (expense)
D. Fear of drug dependence
E. Adverse or side effects
F. Difficulty in obtaining medication
G. Inteference with lifestyle
H. Lack of confidence in physican
I. Lack of proper instruction about medication regimen
J. Other (specify)

INTERVIEW QUESTION	GUIDES AND RATIONALE
20. Where do you store (or keep) your medications?	20. To assess proper storage of medications (e.g., determine if meds requiring refrigeration are stored in refrigerator).
21. When you have problems with or concerns about your medications, do you feel free (comfortable) in calling or talking to your physician?	21. To assess quality of the client/provider relationship. If client does not feel comfortable, additional description of the client/physician relationship should be requested.
22. Is there anyone else you can talk to about your medication concerns? Family, friends, pharmacist?	22. To assess client's choice of support persons regarding medication problems. Are they appropriate (e.g., knowledgeable, reliable) for addressing concerns, giving sound advice?

Reprinted with permission from Susan Guralnick. Model Curriculum Series—Health Beliefs and Medications: Interviewing Techniques. Seattle, Northwest Geriatric Education Center, University of Washington, 1987.

4

Assessment and Management of the Older Patient: A Continuum of Optometric Care

Sheree J. Aston
Joseph H. Maino

An overall perspective of ocular and functional needs must be considered when caring for the elderly patient. Many visual and nonvisual concerns will have to be met by the conclusion of the eye examination. Optometric practitioners should be cognizant of problems that may not be expressed verbally but affect visual performance. Best corrected vision in the office with ideal lighting and print contrast does not necessarily transfer to the home environment. Consider the patient who comes to an optometric office and complains of blurred vision. After a complete evaluation, the patient sees 20/20 at distance and near; however, blurred vision persists with the new glasses. A second visit to the office reveals that the blurred vision occurred when the patient tried to read the newspaper at night in his favorite chair without adequate lighting. In this case, specific questions concerning the exact conditions under which the blurred vision occurred should have been included in the optometric history. It is crucial to understanding the patient symptoms as well as the situation under which vision problems occur in the elderly.

This chapter will focus on the considerations in the evaluation and management of the elderly patient. A continuum of eye-care model is suggested as a guideline for optometric practitioners to individualize the care rendered to older adults. There is variability in the type of care provided to patients, independent of their level of physical, mental, social, and environmental limitations. All patients with chronic physical disabilities are not seen in hospitals or other institutional settings. They may be seen in private offices or in private residences.

Services delivered should be determined by individual patient needs and *not* by the physical setting in which care is given. The functional abilities as well as the visual needs of the elderly need to be explored in any location. The optometric examination cannot be performed without information concerning the functional demands of their "home" environment. The patient should be able to transfer the visual improvement from the optometric office to the home setting. This approach may be applied on successive visits to keep abreast of the changes in visual and functional needs that may have occurred since the previous evaluation.

PATIENT CARE CONTINUUM

Optometric care is given in all types of environments. From least restricted to most restricted, the settings are optometric office or clinic, the private residence, hospital, and long-term care facilities. In providing vision care, the practitioner will deal with older individuals who can be categorized as well, moderately impaired, or severely impaired. Clinicians may encounter well and impaired individuals in traditional and nontraditional settings; optometric services are needed by *all* elderly groups. Following is a description of individuals in these categories and where they are most likely to be found (Mancil and Aston, 1989).

Well Elderly

Well elderly, for the most part, are independent. They may be experiencing chronic health problems but are not functionally impaired. They are however, susceptible to many age-related diseases processes. An important aspect of optometric care is patient education regarding disease that are vision threatening. Older patients need to understand the functional effects of normal vision and aging changes as well as the importance of routine eye examinations. Well elderly can usually be located in senior citizens clubs, centers, life care communities, civic organizations, religious gatherings, and country clubs (Mancil and Aston, 1989).

Moderately Impaired Elderly

Moderately impaired elderly may have the same or more chronic health conditions than the well elderly. The main difference is that this group will more likely need help in performing activities of daily living (i.e., cooking, personal care, shopping). These older adults may also be using assistive devices such as walkers and wheelchairs.

Multiple medication taking among this population is commonplace. It is crucial to ascertain a proper listing of medications and possible side effects that could interfere with visual functioning. The moderately impaired elderly are most likely to be found in senior citizens day care centers, day hospitals, private residences, and life care communities (Mancil and Aston, 1989).

Severely Impaired Elderly

The severely impaired as a segment of the elderly have many more disabling conditions. On the average, they are older and are taking a host of prescribed and over-the-counter medications. It would not be unusual to find various types of "confusion" among this population. The severely impaired geriatric group will most likely be homebound or in a long-term care facility such as a nursing home.

These seniors often will not be able to come to the office for eye care. Usually, severely disabled older persons will require primary, secondary, and perhaps tertiary care. These patients are commonly assessed in private residences (home-bound), hospitals, boarding homes, nursing homes, respite care centers, and skilled nursing facilities of life care communities (Mancil and Aston, 1989).

MODELS FOR VISION CARE

The model in Figure 4-1 should be used to guide the geriatric optometrist through the evaluation process of the impaired older person. It will aid the thought pattern of the practitioner in identifying and managing patient problems. Following the natural flow of this outline will assist the practitioner in determining the patient's problems, ramifications of these problems in everyday life, types of individuals that should be involved in care, as well as the services available to meet individual's challenges and the resources available to provide needed services. Following this plan for care will put into action the key elements of successful networking (Becker, 1985) and guide overall assessment of well, moderately impaired, and severely impaired geriatric individuals. The differences in care of these groups in nontraditional settings is provided at the end of this chapter.

THE OPTOMETRIC EVALUATION

A solid optometric evaluation should begin with a complete history, including ocular and nonocular areas. Data on the medical, social, mental, and functional (nonocular) areas must be collected and assessed (Kane et al., 1989).

Non Visual Assessment

The eye care provider should not expect to evaluate fully nonvisual aspects, but he or she should be able to identify a defect and refer the patient appropriately. A complete history of these areas should be obtained routinely on all elderly patients and the information gathered used to guide the examination or aid patient management decisions. There will be times when all of the data gathered will not be useful for examination purposes; however, the knowledge will serve as a baseline for future evaluations. Always keep in mind, eye care may be the *only* health service an older patient seeks. Optometric referrals for this patient can positively affect overall health care as well as the quality of life. Visual dysfunction may be the result of such underlying problems as clinical depression (see Chapter 10). The relationship of visual symptoms to abnormalities in the nonocular areas must be explored to properly address the patient's problems.

It is recommended that information on the mental, medical, functional, and social areas of the older patient be compiled through the use of preliminary questionnaires, during the history portion of the eye examination, and informally throughout the examination process.

A. Define/diagnose the disease (OD/MD)
   1. Normal vs. abnormal changes
   2. Reversibility–prevention

B. Determine disabilities (OD/MD)
   1. Functional visual and non-visual problems
   2. Possible adaptations–devices, modifications, etc.

C. Ascertain patient needs to be independent/functional (Nurse, OT, PT, O&M, RT)
   1. Rehabilitation
   2. Self-care techniques
   3. Housing
   4. Outside activities
   5. Counseling/therapy
   6. Available help/support

D. Determine which services would meet patient needs (SW)
   1. Geriatric out-patient clinic
   2. Private health care provider
   3. Senior center
   4. Hospital
   5. Adult day care center
   6. Nursing home
   7. In-home health care
   8. In-home personal care
   9. Shopping/transportation service
   10. Friendly visitor service

E. Determine local resources which provide needed services (SW)
   1. Formal–public or private
   2. Informal–family, friends

OD	= Doctor of Optometry	MD	= Doctor of Medicine
OT	= Occupational Therapist	PT	= Physical Therapist
RT	= Rehabilitation Teacher	O&M	= Orientation & Mobility Specialist
SW	= Social Worker		

Figure 4-1 Assessment of the Elderly. (Adapted from Becker MR: Serving the needs of the visually impaired elderly. In Kwitko ML and Weinstock EJ (eds): Geriatric Ophthalmology. Orlando, Grune and Stratton, 1985.)

Mental Status

The mental status of the older patient is an important area of inquiry. An elderly patient who appears confused, paranoid, exhibits inappropriate behavior, or suffers from extreme memory loss should be screened for dementia. A simple useful test for the optometrist to administer is the short portable mental status questionnaire. Basically, it is a list of ten questions that can be administered in 5 to 15 minutes. A copy of the screening test and scoring criteria are included in the Appendix 10-1. Individuals who score low on this test or who exhibit major signs and symptoms identified in Chapter 10 should be referred to their family physician or geriatrician (Warshaw, 1986).

Medical Component

Accurate medical information is an absolute necessity in the evaluation and care of geriatric patients. Most elderly have at least one chronic condition, with many having two or more health problems (Brody, 1986). Consequently, polypharmacy is an area of concern when dealing with the older person. The patient's drug history is extremely important to the care of the aged patient. The patient should be instructed before the actual appointment to bring all medications and prescriptions at the time of the examination. The doctor must ascertain the use of medications and over-the-counter drugs.

In gathering a patient's history, the practitioner must be alert for signs of hearing impairment, confusion, and fatigue. Because elderly patients often present with atypical symptoms of illnesses, be aware of nonspecific complaints such as falling, immobility, mental confusion, urinary incontinence, weakness, changes in eating patterns, and drinking. These symptoms are often a reflection of a chronic illness, as well as a new, life-threatening disease process. Severe headache and chest pain are also examples of nonspecific complaints (Weinstock and Norris, 1985).

The elderly commonly present with nonspecific complaints because of an altered presentation of disease processes. Another reason may be the influence of an acute illness or cognitive impairment. With or without classic symptoms, specific treatable diseases must be ruled out during the examination process (Kane et al., 1989).

An accurate visual health history is, of course, a vital component and is discussed later. Any symptoms of visual problems should be investigated fully (Bailey, 1986).

Functional Abilities

Knowledge of the functional status of the older person is essential to proper patient management. The doctor may know the patient has several chronic conditions yet be unaware of their effect on everyday function. Consider the consequences of a person with arthritis who is unable to open a prescription bottle the practitioner has prescribed for glaucoma.

Assessment of functional abilities involves questioning of the patient's ability to perform independently such activities of daily living as shopping, cooking, self-medication, reading mail, and writing bills (Kane et al., 1989). Optometrists are in a position to refer patients who are unable to care for their personal health and household needs for in-home services.

Social Element

Difficulties in obtaining an accurate history include decreased hearing, mental disorders, and nonspecific symptoms (Kane et al., 1989). The doctor may need to use significant others to ascertain all needed data regarding symptoms the elderly are experiencing.

Understanding the social circumstances of the geriatric patient will assist in meeting his or her needs. It is important to ascertain the living arrangements, lifestyle, and social support systems available to the patient. This will be valuable in the determination of final patient management strategies. It will also improve patient compliance. If the doctor has decided that the older patient is physically unable to self-medicate, it is even more vital to draw upon existing supports. A family member, friend, or perhaps a home health aide may be needed to help with medications.

Importance of NonVisual History

Information on the older patient's nonvisual abilities will be useful in facilitating interdisciplinary care. Optometrists who have obtained preliminary data on these abilities will be able to communicate in a language common to all health practitioners. An understanding of a patient's overall abilities will also enable the optometric practitioner to understand the priority the patient places on the vision problem, and he or she will be able to act accordingly in its management.

The Visual History

The ultimate goal of history taking is to determine the reason for the elderly person's visit to the optometrist's office. It is not uncommon for the older patient to have more than one visual problem. The geriatric patient should be questioned throughout the examination process. Areas of inquiry include problems with driving, reading, television viewing, vision in dim light, glare discomfort, and so on. The patient should be instructed beforehand to bring any assistive devices to the examination, including the best pair of glasses, hearing aids, and dentures. The clinician will be able to communicate better with older patients if they are functioning with their assistive devices (Bailey, 1986; Barressi, 1984).

Considerations in History Taking

A comprehensive history from an older adult can be time-consuming. The doctor frequently is interacting with an elderly patient who is suffering from confusion or a hearing impairment. It is often helpful to use well-directed questions to the person's good (hearing) side. Additional details can be collected from significant others for a person with mild to severe dementia.

The eye care provider should listen carefully to the senior's visual complaints before leading questions or half-answers are offered. In-depth inquiries should be directed around known age-related changes. A well-orchestrated history will ascertain the clinical significance of anomalies such as blepharochalsis, cataract-related myopia, or media opacities (Keeney and Keeney, 1985).

As discussed earlier an important area to investigate is prescribed and non-prescribed drugs. Determine which ones have been prescribed and which are not prescribed (self-medication), when they are taken, what they were originally prescribed for, why any over-the-counter drugs are used, how the drugs are taken, and how they affect visual and overall function.

Ascertain if there is an ocular health problem or mental/social factors that may be related to the patient's vision problems or to a reaction of his vision problems. Try to relate current visual concerns with the information obtained on the nonvisual areas (Barressi, 1985).

Difficulties in History Taking

Communication may be difficult because of reduced vision, hearing, or cognitive function. To overcome these barriers, it is important to have a quiet, well-lit room. Practitioners should speak slowly and in lower tones. The assistive devices for the hearing-impaired person (described in Chapter 9) should be used to facilitate the history and examination. The older patient should be faced directly to allow for lip reading. For the aged adult with mild hearing or vision loss, write questions with a black felt pen in large print on nonglare paper with good contrast. Communication may also be difficult because of diminished normal motor performance. Cognitive function is somewhat slower in older individuals, so it is important for the practitioner to give the patient enough time to respond properly (Kane et al., 1989).

The elderly typically underreport their visual symptoms. Factors involved include individual health beliefs, fear, depression, atypical responses to disease, as well as presence of a confusional state. The practitioner therefore must ask specific questions about suspected symptoms. If the eye care provider is not able to ascertain all the information needed from the patient, relatives, friends, and other care givers will be useful to complete the history (Kane et al., 1989).

Often, there are multiple reasons for visual complaints and the reason for the visit. Older adults may have a health condition that is causing a vision problem, be taking a medication that has an ocular side effect, or have a normal or abnormal vision dysfunction. In the case of multiple problems, the optometrist must deal with each complaint, one at a time. All treatable conditions should be considered and ruled out. All signs and symptoms must be investigated during the examination process. The patient should be interviewed throughout the examination process to get a complete history. As appropriate, screening tests should be administered to gain an understanding of the nonvisual complaints. Any suspected mental or physical diseases or conditions must be referred as soon as possible for full identification and treatment (Kane et al., 1989).

The Ocular Examination

A comprehensive ocular evaluation is crucial to vision care of the geriatric patient. Statistically, the incidence and prevalence of both normal and abnormal changes in the eye increases with age. Care should be taken to access both the external and internal structures of the eye. A slit lamp examination, tonometry, ophthalmoscopy, and visual field should be performed.

During the entire examination process, eye care professionals should explain the procedures being performed and why. This type of education is particularly critical during the ocular health portion of the evaluation. Geriatric patients are typically concerned about conditions such as cataracts and glaucoma. In fact, the elderly may be harboring secret fears about vision-threatening conditions. These fears are often not expressed to the doctor who is often viewed as an authority figure. It is the responsibility of the practitioner to inform the patient regarding the status of their ocular health and to address the importance of regular and timely examinations (Bailey, 1986).

Visual Acuity and Glare

Acuity testing should be performed under normal and low illumination (Anan, 1989). Visual acuity (VA) may be enhanced by use of low vision charts or new charts of variable contrasting, including those by Bailey and Pelli. These charts enable acuity to be recorded and estimated under a variety of contrasting conditions. Mentor, BVAT, Arden gratings, and Vistech contrast sensitivity test are useful in diagnosing patients with cataracts and glaucoma. It also helps to explain nonspecific complaints. If the patient presents with multiple pairs of spectacles, test acuity through the ones most frequently worn. Always test with a pinhole occluder to see if the patient's VA will improve (Mancil, 1989).

Testing for glare helps to quantify the patient's amount of glare disability or discomfort. Glare disturbances may be one of the early symptoms of a media opacity. The Mentor, BAT, IRAS, interferometry glare tester, and the Titmus Glare Tester are recommended to test for glare disability (Mancil, 1989).

Refraction

Refraction of the older patient may be more difficult due to smaller pupils and cloudy media. Furthermore, the refraction itself may take more time to complete. Again, the optometrist should leave adequate time for response from the older patient. Refraction is an important technique, considering almost all older adults have some type of refractive error. Both objective and subjective methods can be used. Although many older patients can be refracted with phoroptor, one of the authors (JHM) finds the use of the trial frame much quicker and more reliable. Retinoscopy techniques may need to be modified because of miotic pupils and nontransparent media. Elderly patients with small pupils may be dilated to enhance the refraction. If this is not possible, try performing retinoscopy at a closer working distance (radical retinoscopy) to help maximize the retinal reflex. In radical retinoscopy, a working lens is subtracted from the final result and then is modified accordingly to the working distance. The observation of the brightness and clarity of the retinal reflex will give the doctor valuable information on the elderly patient's ocular condition. Subjective refraction requires brighter light, greater contrast, and more substantial trial lens changes. The subjective retinoscopy should be performed using a greater "just noticeable difference" than normally used (Barressi, 1985, Mancil, 1989; Mancil, 1990).

A high contrast VA chart should be used during the refraction. A greater dioptric change should be used in evaluating the cylindrical correction. A handheld Jackson Cross Cylinder (JCC) with 0.50 diopter changes or higher is recommended. The hand-held JCC can be held in front of the phoropter if it cannot be modified in place of a built-in JCC (Mancil, 1990).

The trial frame refraction is the best refraction technique to use for aphakic and low vision patients. (Refer to Chapter 7 for more information on trial frame refraction.) A correct vertex distance is vital for aphakic patients. Reduced test distances may increase the accuracy and sensitivity of the older patients' responses. Another method to consider is trial lens clip over the patient's existing prescription. After completion of the over refraction, the spectacles with a lens clips and trial lenses are placed in a lensometer and the back vertex power is measured. Any refraction that is significantly different from the patient's habitual prescription should be trial framed (Bailey, 1986).

Ocular Health Assessment

Due to an increased incidence of such age-related disorders as cataract, macular degeneration, glaucoma, and diabetic retinopathy, all older patients need a careful ocular health assessment. After determining the patient's visual acuity, check pupillary responses. Keep in mind that erroneous findings may occur as a consequence of age-related or drug-induced miosis or past ocular surgery or trauma. A "reverse" swinging flashlight test or a "subjective" brightness test* may be needed to determine if an optic nerve abnormality is present.

Older patients can also exhibit problems with binocular vision. Diplopia may occur due to a breakdown of a high phoria, a previous cerebral vascular accident (CVA), or secondary to trauma. Do a cover/uncover test at distance and near. Make sure to test through the patient's bifocal correction when evaluating the patient at near. Also check the patient's ocular motility by having him or her fixate and follow a penlight through the primary positions of gaze.

A visual field evaluation should be done if the patient complains or history warrants it. Amsler grid testing should be done if the patient notes a central scotoma or distorted vision. If the patient has a history of CVA, take the time to do a confrontation visual field. You may be surprised at what you find!

Goldman perimetric visual fields or automated fields should be done on those older patients who can tolerate the procedure. Pay particular attention to patient comfort. Check the back support on the chair and provide adequate break points.

Evaluation of the eye and adnexa should begin with a gross penlight inspection. Note the lid margins. Is there good apposition of the lids and globe? Does the patient have an extropion or entropion? Does the patient have a chronic blepharitis or meibomianitis? Is a corneal reflex present? Is the conjunctiva clear? Pull down the lower lid. Are symnblephoran present? Evert the upper lid. Note any scarring.

After this gross inspection, perform biomicroscopy. Again, pay attention to patient positioning. If he or she is kyphotic or exhibits some other skeletal defor-

---

*The eye with the optic nerve defect will have a diminished brightness sense when compared to the normal eye.

mity, you may need to use a hand-held slit lamp. If a hand-slit lamp is not available, use a +20D binocular indirect opthalmoscopy condensing lens or +20D hand-held magnifier and an external light source to view the anterior segment.

During biomicroscopy be sure to note the quality and quantity of the tear film. Although ocular surface disease is not typically a sight-threatening disorder, it can produce intermittent blur and irritation. To minimize these symptoms, prescribe the appropriate tear substitute. Make sure to treat adequately any concomitant blepharitis or meibomianitis.

While examining the anterior segment estimate the angle depth and note any cell or flare. Evaluate the iris for rubeosis. After the pupil is dilated, evaluate the lens for nuclear sclerosis, cortical changes, and posterior subcapsular opacities. For pseudophakes assess the position and stability of the intraocular lens. Also note any posterior capsular fibrosis that is present. The optic nerve and macula may be evaluated with a 90 or 78D lens at this time as well.

Because older patients are at greater risk for glaucoma, Goldmann tonometry should always be done. If the patient is unable to be positioned in the slit lamp for Goldmann's tonometry, use a hand-held instrument such as the tonopen or Perkins' tonometer.

All geriatric patients should have a baseline dilated fundus evaluation. Those patients with gonoscopically verified narrow angles should be counseled concerning the possibility of an acute glaucoma attack. If the patient consents to the evaluation, dilate one eye to determine if the pressure increases. This provocative test should be done early in the day if possible. (Bartlett & Jannus 1989) Obviously, if the intraocular pressure rises, treat appropriately* and refer for a laser peripheral iridectomy when the patient is stable.

There are many tools (BIO, 90D lens, 78D lens, Hruby lens) to help in the evaluation of the posterior pole. When deciding on which diagnostic procedures to use keep in mind the physical limitations of the patient. For example, it may be difficult to incline the patient for indirect ophthalmoscopy if severe chronic obstructive pulmonary disease is present. Adapt the procedures to meet each patient's needs.

EYE CARE IN NONTRADITIONAL SETTINGS

The number of oldest of the old and disabled elderly will continue to grow into the twenty-first century. A correspondingly increasing number of elderly will require eye care in hospital settings, long-term care facilities, and their family residencies. Optometrists must be prepared to provide quality eye care in both traditional and nontraditional settings.

A full complement of specific equipment is recommended for examining the older patient, especially those disabled, regardless of setting. Equipment includes

---

*Initital treatment includes the use of topical pilocarpine or a beta blocker and when necessary, orally administered acetazolamide. (Bartlett & Jannus, 1989)

the biomicroscope, binocular indirect ophthalmoscope, 20D, 60D, and 90D condensing lenses, goniolens, three-mirror lens, and diagnostic kit. Retinoscopy bars, trial frames and lenses, VA charts (such as the Feinbloom VA chart), Genelli or Halberg clips, and hand held CCs will be needed for refraction. Portable hand-held equipment such as Schiotz tonometer, hand-held tonometer (Perkins or Kowan and Tonopen), hand-held slit lamp, portable Goldmann tonometer, and hand-held lensometer are recommended. Additional equipment such as a comfortable stool, portable tangent screen, extension cord, black out drape, and third-party provider forms are suggested (Swanson, 1990).

Home Eye Care

Advanced preparation for in-home and long-term care will decrease the evaluation time in these settings. A clinical data sheet should be completed with the patient's address, telephone number, age, and pertinent history. Before making a home visit, attempt to get a history on the patient, including needs and expectations. The patient, a family member, or home health worker may provide this information. Existing ocular and medical records should be requested to assist in the examination. All of the suggested portable equipment should be available for the examination itself (Anstice, 1986).

Homebound elderly are usually either recuperating from an acute hospitalizing illness or are suffering from chronic debilitating diseases but have been able to delay institutionalization. The ultimate goal of care of a homebound patient is to encourage independence. In addition to providing the best VA possible, optometrists must consider improving the patient's visual functioning through modification of environmental lighting and contrast (Swanson, 1990).

Successful home care programs can be aided by a local area agency on aging, home health care agencies, visiting nurses programs, and hospital discharge planners. Keep in mind that medicare reimbursement for home visits are similar to those allowed for office visits. Actually, this may be impractical for the clinician. The alternative is to set the home visit fee commensurate with the examination time, time away from the office, and additional staff time. This would, of course, calculate at several times the cost of a private office visit. In actuality, most optometrists provide home services at their office visit fee structure. The difference in reimbursement is often outweighed by the satisfaction gained in helping these homebound patients. Improved vision function can greatly improve the life satisfaction of the impaired elderly. There are other tangible benefits such as networking with other health care providers, which may increase referrals to the private office practice (Swanson, 1990; Mancil, 1989).

Nursing Home Care

The vast majority of geriatric individuals reside with their family, spouse, or alone in private homes; however, at any point in time, 1.5 million seniors, or 5% of the elderly population live in nursing homes. Over a lifetime, 20% to 60%

of persons 65 years of age and older will reside in a nursing home before they expire (Howe et al., 1986; Swanson, 1990). The population in a nursing home is significantly different than a noninstitutionalized patient base. The institutionalized adult has a greater chance of suffering from a confusional state. This population, furthermore, commonly suffers from a vision impairment. The incidence of vision disabilities among long-term care patients has been estimated to range between 19% and 35% (Swanson, 1990). Dementia among long-term care residents have been estimated to affect as many as 50% (Kane et al., 1989). These patients may be ambulatory, wheelchair-confined or bedridden.

The equipment suggested for nursing home visits is the same as for home visits. In case of a very large nursing home, the practitioner may consider the set-up of a permanent lane. In addition to basic equipment, low vision devices and testing equipment are recommended for this population. A variety of microscopes and telescopes of varying powers is suggested. Vision care provided at nursing homes may be more financially feasible for the average practitioner than the home visit program. Most of the elderly patients will be covered both by medicare and medicaid, but it is overwhelming a medicaid versus medicare-financed program. A good number of patients also have other third-party insurance. Nursing home care may be even more lucrative because, if scheduled properly, the clinician may examine a multitude of patients in one day.

Important contacts at long-care facilities are the social worker, nursing home administrator, and head nurse. The nursing home administrator is usually the person who will decide whether the optometric practitioner may perform examinations at the facility. The initial contact should therefore be with the nursing home administrator for contracted services. The staff physician then will decide the type of duties the optometrist may perform within the facility. Typically, the attending physician controls the patient's overall health care. A good working relationship with the staff physician is needed for the optometrist to manage patients properly. Good sources of information about the patients' problems are the nurses or the nursing assistants. They can provide specific information on visual complaints and needs (Swanson, 1990; Anstice, 1986).

REFERENCES

Anan B. Understanding the older patient. Optometric Manage, Nov 1989; 38–42.

Anstice J. Vision in the home and in institutional settings. In Rosenbloom AA, Morgan MW (eds): Vision and Aging, general and clinical perspectives. New York, Professional Prepbooks/Fairchild Publications, 1986.

Bailey IL. The optometric examination of the elderly patient. In Rosenbloom AA, Morgan MW (eds): Vision and aging, general and clinical perspectives, New York, Professional Press Books/Fairchild Publications, 1986, pp 189–209.

Barresi B: Optometric assessment of the aged—general principles. In Rosenbloom A (ed): Workbook on Optometric Gerontology: Washington, American Optometric Association, 1985.

Bartlett J, Jannus S. Clinical Ocular Pharmacology. Butterworths, Boston, 1989.

Becker MR. Serving the needs of visually impaired elderly. In Kwitko ML, Weinstock FJ (eds): Geriatric Ophthalmology. Orlando, Grune and Stratton, 1985, pp 15–29.

Brody S. Aging, Disability and Therapeutic Optimism. *In* Brody S, Russ G (eds): Aging and Rehabilitation. New York, Springer Publishing, 1986.

Howe AL, Phillips C, Preston GA. Analyzing access to nursing home care. Soc Sci Med 1986;23:1267–77.

Kane RL, Ouslander JG, Abrass JB. Evaluating the elderly patient. *In* Essentials of Clinical Geriatrics. New York, McGraw Hill, 1989, pp 47–78.

Keeney VT, Keeney AH. Emotional aspects of visual impairment in the population over 60 years of age. *In* Kwitko ML, Weinstock FJ (eds): Geriatric Ophthalmology. Orlando, Grune and Stratton, 1985.

Mancil GL. Optometric evaluation and management of the well older adult. *In* Aston SJ, DeSylvia DA, Mancil GL (eds): Optometric Gerontology: A Resource Manual for Educators. Rockville, American Association of Schools of Optometry, 1989.

Mancil GL. Serving the needs of older patients through private practice settings. Optom Vis Sci May 1990; 67(5):315–318.

Mancil GL, Aston SJ. Community health issues in optometric gerontology. *In* Aston SJ, DeSylvia DA, Mancil GL (eds): Optometric Gerontology: A Resource Manual for Educators. Rockville, American Association of Schools and Colleges of Optometry, 1989, pp 10–14.

Swanson MW. Optometric care of the homebound an institutionalized older adult. Optom Vis Sci 1990;67(5):323–328.

Warshaw GA. Management of cognitive impairment in the elderly. New Dev Med Sep 1986;1(2)40–53.

Weinstock FJ, Norris JW. Approach to and examination of the geriatric patient. *In* Kwitko ML, Weinstock FJ (eds): Geriatric Ophthalmology. Orlando, Grune and Stratton, 1985.

5

Normal Vision Problems of the Elderly

Mary Jo Horn
Joseph H. Maino

The elderly portion of our population is growing rapidly, and the importance of understanding the aging visual system is obvious. A fine line often separates normal aging changes from ocular disease. This chapter focuses on the healthy older adult eye and the effects the normal aging process has on the image-forming system and the neurosensory system, as well as the impact normal aging has on various visual functions.

TEAR FILM

The tear film is important for maintenance of the smooth, regular refractive surface of the cornea and to the health of the anterior surface of the conjunctiva and cornea. The tear film loses stability with increasing age. The stability of the tear film depends on both the quantity and the quality of the components of the tear film as well as on the blinking process (Patel and Farrell, 1989).

Because of the inherent problems that exist with the measurement of the tears, quantifying tear production is difficult; however, authors agree that lacrimation decreases with increasing age (Paschides, 1991; Hamano et al, 1990; de Roeth, 1953; Henderson and Prough, 1950). Using a modified Schirmer's test, de Roeth (1953) found that the tear production at age 40 is approximately one half of that found in the first decade of life. He noted that it continues to decline slowly until the values at age 80 are one fourth to one fifth those found in the first decade of life (Table 5-1). To assess the effect of age on the tear film stability, Patel and Farrell (1989) looked at the tear thinning time (TTT) for observers between the ages of 8 and 80 years. The TTT is similar in concept to the commonly used break up time (BUT), but the TTT was used because it did not require the instillation of fluorescein, which is thought to reduce the stability of the tear film. These researchers found that the TTT declines significantly with age. The results show that the TTT is reduced by at least one half from age 8 to age 80 years. Changes in

51

Table 5-1 Lacrimation Measured with Modified Schirmer Test in Various Age Groups

Age	Male Tear Production	No. of Eyes	Female Tear Production	No. of Eyes
6–9	63	12	63.8	19
10–19	59	70	63.4	60
20–29	40.8	44	47.4	39
30–39	41.2	33	34.2	47
40–49	31.1	42	38.8	80
50–59	22.8	34	26.4	79
60–69	21.4	44	23.9	82
70–79	16.2	32	17.4	72
80+	11.5	15	16	22

From de Roetth A: Lacrimation in normal eyes. Arch Ophthalmol 49:185–189, 1953. Used with permission.

the aqueous, the oily, and to a lesser extent the mucin layer, of the tear film have all been implicated in this decrease of stability.

Benedetto et al. (1984), in their studies of the blinking process, found that forceful blinking can increase tear film thickness. An increase in thickness can help provide for a more adequate tear volume. Conversely, a weaker than normal blink should produce the opposite effect. Thus, they speculate that the older eyelid, as it experiences some senile relaxation of its elastic structure, should have a weaker and less efficient blink.

Clinically, the older patient may express concern with short-term visual fluctuations, especially with tasks requiring increased concentration (refraction, reading, driving, and so on). The average person blinks spontaneously 15 to 20 times per minute. During tasks requiring more concentration, the blink rate may go down to as little as 3 or 4 blinks per minute (Milder, 1987). The reduction in the tear film stability, especially when combined with a reduction in the blink rate with concentration, may be a source of irritation or frustration for the older patient. Educating the patient on the need to blink more, the use of tear supplements and lid hygiene may help to minimize this phenomenon.

CORNEA

A clear cornea is important for the production of a sharp image on the retina. Fortunately, the transparency of the cornea does not appear to be affected greatly by the normal aging process (Marmor, 1986). Optically, the anterior surface of the cornea must be kept smooth and moist. The eyelid and the tear film share this responsibility.

The clearness of the cornea is attributed mostly to the uniformly small diameter (approximately 300Å) and close spacing (approximately 550Å) of the stromal collagen fibrils and other smaller corneal cells (Klyce and Beuerman, 1988). According to Goldman et al. (1968), light scatter and thus loss of transparency should be minimal in the healthy cornea because of its relatively small refractive elements (less than 2000Å) in comparison to the wavelength of light (approximately 5000Å). Clarity may be lost if this functional structure of the cornea is altered as in corneal edema, injury, and disease.

One of the primary functions of the endothelium is to maintain proper corneal dehydration (Dohlman, 1983). This is important to the health and the clarity of the cornea. The corneal endothelium is a single layer of cells that is, for the most part, amitotic after birth. (Mitosis of human endothelium has been demonstrated in tissue culture from young corneas [Waring et al., 1982].) The cells, however, have the ability to enlarge and spread out postnatally and during cell loss secondary to aging to help preserve normal visual function. The endothelium has 3500 to 4000 cells/mm² at birth. This cell density drops to between 1400 to 2500 cells/mm² in the adult cornea (Klyce and Beuerman, 1988). The endothelial cell count may be as low as 900 cells/mm² in the ninth decade of life (Waring et al., 1982). The endothelium is able to maintain proper dehydration until the cell count drops to the critical level of 400 to 700 cells/mm² (Klyce and Beuerman, 1988). Thus, the healthy aging cornea should be expected to maintain transparency throughout life.

PUPIL

Pupil size decreases with age. The average dark-adapted pupillary diameter decreases between the ages of 20 and 80 by about 2.5 mm (Birren et al., 1950; Loewenfeld, 1979). The exact cause of the reduction in pupil size is not known; however several mechanisms have been suggested. Atrophy of the dilator muscle fibers and thus loss of their contractile ability is considered a causative factor. Along with this apparent decrease in muscle function, authors also mention a variety of age-related degenerative structural changes in the iris and/or its vascular supply (Morgan, 1986; Kline and Schieber, 1985). Aging changes in the innervation of the iris muscles is another popular theory. A third possible explanation offered and elaborated on by Loewenfeld (1979) is that of defective central inhibition. Regardless of the cause of the decrease in pupil size, it is thought to contribute to the age-related reduction in retinal illuminance.

The reduction in the amount of light entering the eye may contribute to decreased visual function in the elderly. The role of the pupil as it relates to this will be discussed in the appropriate visual function sections later. One presumed advantage of the smaller pupil is that it helps decrease on the size of the blur circle when the eye is not in focus, and with this, the depth of focus is apparently improved (Moses, 1987; Weale, 1963). Interestingly, Morgan (1986) feels the reduced blur circle size may make subjective refractions more difficult in older patients. He concludes that the relative lack of critical sensitivity to lens changes during refractions may be more related to pupil size and the optics of the eye than to poor patient observation skills.

LENS

The density of the ocular media increases with age. The crystalline lens is considered the major factor in this age-related change (Werner et al., 1990). A decrease in transmissivity with age occurs in both the visible and the ultraviolet (UV) regions of the spectrum (Weale, 1988). An increase in the crystalline lens absorption produces an age-related decrease in retinal illumination. Weale (1963), noting a decrease in the quantity as well as the spectral quality of light reaching the retina, concluded that the amount of light reaching the retina of a 60-year old is only one third the amount of light that reaches the retina of a 20-year old. He attributes most of the loss to the lens, with the pupil playing a lesser role.

The age-related change in the density of the lens is considered to be linear up to about age 60 years (Werner et al., 1990). Nonlinearity is noted by some researchers after the age of 60 years. In their review of this subject, Pokorny et al. (1987) noted a three-fold change in the rate of increase in the optical density of the lens after the age of 60 years (0.12 density unit per decade at 400 nm between ages 20 to 60 years and 0.40 density unit per decade above age 60 years). Werner et al. (1990), however, pointed out the possible ambiguity in the separation of cataractous subjects from noncataractous subjects in this older patient population.

The age-related change in the spectral density and the yellowing of the lens have been attributed to the increase in lens thickness and/or to the deposition of pigment. The lens grows slowly throughout life. Equatorially, new cells are continually produced, with the older cells being compacted toward the center of the encapsulated lens. At birth the axial diameter of the lens is approximately 3.5 to 4.0 mm and increases to approximately 5.0 mm by age 80 years (Tripathi and Tripathi, 1983). Mellerio (1971) found that the lenticular pigment distribution remains unchanged between ages 20 and 60 years. He concluded that the increase in the lenticular yellowing must be accredited solely to the increase in lens thickness. Mellerio's conclusion was challenged by several authors, and in a second paper (1987) he stands strongly by his original conclusion. Lerman (1983) reports that chronic UV exposure over an individual's lifetime induces a photochemical generation and accumulation of at least two chromophores (which absorb at 360 nm and 435 nm and fluoresce at 440 nm and 520 nm, respectively). He believes that as the lens ages the fluorescent compounds increase in concentration, and this results in a progressive decrease in the transmission of visible and UV light with a concomitant increase in the yellow color of the lens. Weale (1988) briefly mentions the addition of a chromophore in his discussion of transmittance of the lens but implies that the phenomenon is mostly due to the increase in the lens thickness. Others (Zigman, 1978; Tan cited in Pokorny, 1987) believe that both the lens growth and pigmentation are involved in the change in the spectral density and yellowing of the lens.

NEURAL CHANGES

Researchers agree that optical factors alone cannot account for the functional visual changes that accompany the normal aging process (Weale, 1975; Morrison and McGrath, 1985; Werner et al., 1990). Neural changes have been implicated as significant factors in the age-related decline in visual function. Age-related degenerative changes and cell loss from the retina to the visual cortex support this view.

With age the retina experiences a variety of changes that some researchers believe may help contribute to the functional decline in the visual system. The number of retinal pigment epithelial (RPE) cells in the posterior pole decreases significantly with age (Dorey et al., 1989). Dorey et al. also studied the accumulation of RPE lipofuscin with age, and correlated this age-related change to a decrease in the number of photoreceptors. Gartner and Henkind (1981) noted a displacement and loss of photoreceptor nuclei from the outer nuclear layer (ONL) with increasing age; along with the loss of cells in the ONL and found a similar reduction in the quantity of the attached rods and cones and the outer plexiform layer axons. Marshall et al. (1979), in a similar study, found an increased incidence in convoluted rod outer segments with increasing age.

Age appears to have an effect on the number of retinal ganglion cell axons in the optic nerve (Tsai et al., 1992; Repka and Quigley, 1989; Balazsi et al., 1984). Balazsi et al. (1984) estimate that a 70-year-old optic nerve has lost approximately 25% of its axons (at a rate of 5637 axons per year). The implications for loss of at least some visual transmission from the retina to the lateral geniculate nucleus are obvious. At a higher level an even more substantial loss is noted. In the macular projection area of the visual cortex, Devaney and Johnson (1980) report a cell loss of almost 50% from age 20 years to age 80 years (46 million neurons per gram of tissue at age 20 to about 24 million neurons per gram at age 80). In addition to the quantitative loss, the quality of the surviving neurons may also suffer (Scheibel et al., 1975).

REFRACTION AND ACCOMMODATION

A trend toward hyperopia (less myopia) exists after age 40 years (Exford 1965; Lavery et al., 1988). This progression of the hyperopia lies somewhere between + 0.25D and + 0.50D per decade (Slataper, 1950; Hirsch, 1959; Exford, 1965). After age 70 years the trend appears to reverse, and a slight shift toward myopia may be noted (Slataper, 1950; Lavery et al., 1988).

There is a clear switch with age from with-the-rule astigmatism to against-the-rule astigmatism (Saunders, 1988). The astigmatic power change with age is not as clearly documented. Most studies reveal little if any cylinder power change with increasing age (Slataper, 1950; Exford, 1965; Saunders, 1988; Lavery et al.,

1988); however, Hirsch (1959) did document an increase in cylinder power with age.

Several studies have been done comparing the accuracy of retinoscopy with subjective refraction. In an age-related comparative study Millodot and O'Leary (1978) confirmed the finding that there is an underestimation of myopia in younger subjects by 0.3D to 0.4D. This discrepancy gradually diminishes as the subjects age, and by age 50 years the situation reverses to a slight overestimation of myopia with retinoscopy.

The amplitude of accommodation gradually decreases with age (Figure 5-1, Moses, 1987). In determining the cause for this reduction, both the lens and the ciliary muscle have been considered. Most authors agree that the decline can be attributed to aging changes related to the lens (Fisher, 1973; Moses, 1987). Studies of the ciliary muscle reveal that the movement required by the muscle fibers per diopter of accommodation is not altered by the aging process (Swegmark, 1969 as cited in Fisher, 1973; Moses 1987).

VISUAL ACUITY

Visual acuity (VA) in the healthy aging eye begins to change around age 50 (Figure 5-2) (Weale, 1975; Pitts, 1982). Resolution depends on the quality of the image presented to the retina, the integrity of the retina, and the neural capacity. In addition to the normal change in VA, the incidence of eye disease with sight-threatening potential rises with age.

The two factors most often noted as having an adverse affect on the image quality are the pupil and the lens. Weale (1975) states that the effect of senile miosis on acuity in the light-adapted eye is small. He also notes that the senile reduction in acuity is unlikely to be due only to the pupil and to the effect of the aging lens.

The role of the aging lens was evaluated by Jay et al. (1987). They assessed visual acuity in 111 patients who had undergone uncomplicated extracapsular cataract extraction and in 50 patients who underwent uncomplicated intracapsular

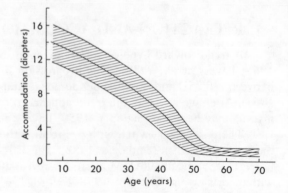

Figure 5-1 Amplitude of accommodation as it varies with age. *From* Duane, A. *Arch Opthalmology.* 54:568, 1928.

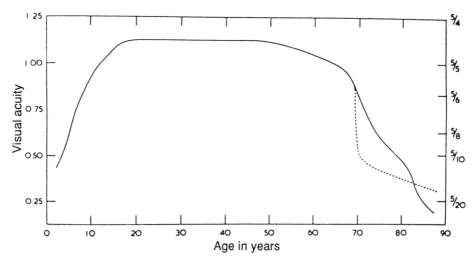

Figure 5-2 Visual acuity as a function of age. The dotted line indicates the acuity in patients with cataracts. *From* Pitts DG. The effects of aging on selected visual functions: Dark adaptation, visual acuity, stereopsis, and brightness contrast. *In* Sekuler R, Kline D, Dismukes K (eds): Aging and Human Visual Function. New York, Alan R. Liss, 1982.

cataract extraction (10–23 years prior to evaluation). Their results indicate that the best corrected acuity after cataract removal declines by 1 line per 13.4 years from 6/5 at age 50 years to around 6/12 at age 90 years. The relationship between VA and age was identical when comparing the extracapsular patients with the intracapsular patients. Thus the authors feel that the results have little to do with the postsurgical status of their subjects. The postsurgical results show a similar trend to the decline noted by Morrison and McGrath (1985) in 20 phakic subjects evaluated with laser interferometry. These findings support the view of Weale (1975) that the neurosensory components are responsible for most of the age-related decline in VA and not the crystalline lens.

CONTRAST SENSITIVITY

Contrast sensitivity function (CSF) is considered to be a more comprehensive assessment of visual function than VA (Elliot, 1987). Older adults show deterioration of contrast sensitivity (Figure 5-3) at higher spatial frequencies (Morrison and McGrath, 1985; Elliott, 1987; Owsley, 1985; Werner et al., 1990; Elliott et al., 1990; Adachi-Usami, 1990). The principal cause for the reduction of this visual function has been the subject of much debate. Increased lenticular absorption and scatter and reduction of retinal illuminance from the miotic pupil in the aging eye have been considered viable explanations (Owsley, 1985; Wright and Drasdo, 1985). Current research, however, indicates that the lens and the pupil have little

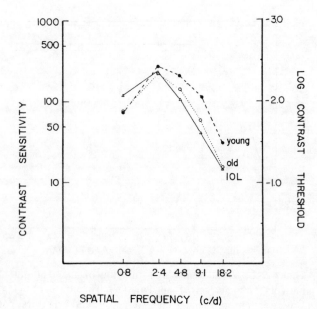

Figure 5-3 Contrast sensitivity loss noted in older phakic and pseudophakic observers. *From* Owsley, C, et al. Role of the crystalline lens in the spatial vision loss of the elderly. *Invest Opthalmol Vis Sci,* 1985; 26:1165–70.

to no effect on the CSF and that the changes are attributable to neuron loss within the visual pathway. Adachi-Usami (1990), Owsley (1985), and Morrison and McGrath (1985) have compared CSF in phakic and pseudophakic eyes. They are in agreement that the reduction in function is neural and conclude that the lens has little to no influence on the CSF. Other researchers (Elliott et al., 1990) have used neutral density filters with young observers in an attempt to simulate the aging lens. Again, the conclusion that the lens has no significant impact on the sensitivity.

The pupil has also been the subject of considerable research on this topic. Miotics (Elliott et al., 1990) have been used, as well as artificial pupils and mydriatics to help determine the role of the pupil in the decreased CSF. Morrison and McGrath (1985), Werner et al. (1990), Elliott et al. (1990) and others agree that the pupil is not a major factor in the loss of contrast with age.

COLOR VISION

Color discrimination progressively declines with increasing age (Cooper et al., 1991, Roy et al., 1991; Knoblauch et al., 1987). The color spectrum is not uniformally affected by age. A tritan-like color defect is observable in patients over age 60 (Roy et al., 1991; Knoblauch et al., 1987; Verriest et al., 1982). The change is attributed to the changes in absorption of the ocular media and to the receptor and/or postreceptor pathways (Werner and Steele, 1988).

Age affects the intensity and spectral distribution of the retinal stimulus. A reduction in pupil size, along with the increase in absorption by the crystalline lens, combine to weaken the stimulus received by the retina (Cooper et al., 1991). Werner et al. (1990) point out that the smaller pupil not only reduces the amount of light that enters the eye, but also directs the light through the thickest portion of the crystalline lens. Verriest (1963), using short wavelength absorbing filters, simulated in the young the tritan-like age-related color vision loss on the Farnsworth-Munsell 100 hue test. When using the Farnsworth-Munsell 100 hue test, Knoblauch et al. (1987) noted that the effects of aging on performance were similar to those found in young observers when illuminance levels were lowered. They found that 20- to 40-year olds at 5.7lx behave similarly to 50- to 60-year olds between 18lx and 57lx and like 70-year olds at 180lx. Knoblauch et al. (1987) believe that the effects of lower illuminance levels on the Farnsworth-Munsell 100 hue test may be related to the Bezold-Brucke effect. This effect refers to the role that intensity plays in hue perception. The blue/yellow components are thought to be the more prominent portion of the stimulus at higher levels of intensity, whereas the red/green components are more dominant at lower intensities.

Three classes of cones are responsible for normal color vision: short-wavelength-sensitive (SWS), medium-wavelength-sensitive (MWS), and long-wavelength-sensitive (LWS). All three classes of cones are thought to decline in sensitivity with age (Werner et al., 1990; Werner and Steele, 1988; Johnson et al., 1988). The SWS cones appear to be more affected by the age-related changes in the ocular media than the MWS and the LWS cones. Werner and Steele (1988), in agreement with Johnson et al. (1988), believe that 40% or more of the SWS loss is attributable to the ocular media. The remaining loss is secondary to receptoral and/or postreceptoral changes.

MWS and LWS cones are more difficult to isolate and study due to their greater spectral sensitivity overlap. Knowledge of these cones is less extensive than knowledge of the SWS cones. Werner and Steele (1988) found similar age-related rates of sensitivity decline in the SWS, MWS, and LWS cones. They point out that the MWS and LWS cones must exhibit more of their age-related change at the receptoral and/or postreceptoral level because the ocular media apparently reduces the short wavelengths more than the longer wavelengths.

DARK ADAPTATION

Older patients often express concern about the reduction in their ability to function in poorly illuminated surroundings. Studies of dark adaptation clearly demonstrate a significant rise in threshold with increasing age (Figure 5-4) (Robertson and Yudkin, 1944; Domey et al., 1960; Eisner et al., 1987).

The decline in sensitivity is due to media and neural changes. Aging changes in the lens and the pupil are considered to be more detrimental to this function than neural changes. In fact, Pitts (1982) states that "the data demonstrate overwhelmingly that losses in ocular transmittance and pupillary miosis resulting from the aging process are sufficient to account for most of

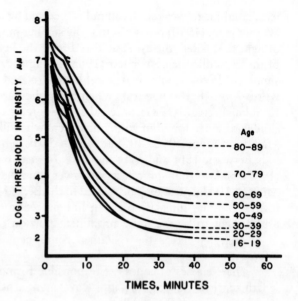

Figure 5-4 Dark adaptation as a function of age. *From* Domey RG, McFarland RA, Chadwick E. Threshold and rate of dark adaptation as functions of age and time. *Hum Factors* 1960; Aug:109–120.

the loss in adaptation, and that only a small portion of the total effect can be attributed to other causes."

VISUAL FIELDS

Visual fields (VF) can provide the clinician with valuable information, but the age of the patient must be considered when analyzing results. An age-related linear decline in the sensitivity of the VF has been noted for both kinetic and static perimetry. Kinetic testing reveals a decrease in the size of the VF of 1° to 3° per decade (Werner, 1991). The mean sensitivity for the static testing shows a reduction of 0.5 dB to 1.0 dB per decade (Jaffe et al., 1986; Haas et al., 1986; Werner, 1991). The peripheral VF apparently declines at a faster rate than the central VF. Jaffe et al. (1986) state that the rate of decline is approximately twice as fast at 30° from fixation than directly at fixation. They go on to say that the reason for the more rapid peripheral decline is not known, but they speculate that the decline is related to the lower concentration of neural elements representing the peripheral VF relative to those representing the central VF. Consequently, when neural loss does occur it is more readily apparent in peripheral testing.

Age may also have an impact on the variability of VF testing over time. Katz and Sommer (1987) performed VF testing three times on healthy subjects over an average period of 18 months. The intervals between the successive VFs was chosen to simulate the frequencies at which VFs might be performed clinically. For patients in the under age 60 group they found the mean SD to be 1.9 dB (range 1.2–2.8 dB) and in the over age 60 group the mean SD was 4.8 dB (range 2.2–8.3dB). The areas of greatest variability were in the periphery and in the superior VF. The variability observed among older subjects over time may cloud the clinical picture.

Age changes in the VF are most likely due to a form of neurosensory loss (Haas et al., 1986; Jaffe et al., 1986). Researchers have attempted to eliminate the optical effects of lens changes, as well as pupil diameter, in their studies by careful patient selection (Jaffe et al., 1986). A pupil size of less than 2.5 mm may have a deleterious effect on the VF because of the reduction of retinal illuminance (Werner, 1991; Lynn et al., 1989) and because of a reduction of the resolving power of the eye that may result from diffraction at the pupil border (Lynn et al., 1989). This effect might be particularly pronounced in the glaucoma patient on miotics but should not influence the visual field results of the healthy aging eye.

SUMMARY

Life means change. This chapter has described how the visual system changes over time. Remember that individuals do not all age in exactly the same way nor do individual body parts or systems age at the same rate. Each of us is unique. One individual may exhibit cataractous changes, whereas another may have perfectly clear lenses but experience some macular changes.

As a group, older adults tend to accept the aging process well. Many even *expect* to move a little slower, hear a little less, and take a little more medicine. However, it's interesting to note that these same individuals are not always as accepting of even small changes in vision—when new glasses are prescribed, they expect to see better. Consequently, it's important to discuss the normal age-related vision changes with patients before they receive their new spectacle prescription. Let the patient watch educational videos which explain and define the common vision problems associated with aging. Provide the patient with pamphlets that describe illumination requirements, tips on driving, and so on. If your patients know what to expect, they will be able to maximize their vision and lead more comfortable and fulfilling lives.

REFERENCES

Adachi-Usami, E. Senescence of visual function as studied by visually evoked cortical potentials. Jpn J Ophthalmol 1990; 34:81–94.

Balazsi AG, Bootman J, Drance SM, et al. The effect of age on the nerve fiber population of the human optic nerve. Am J Ophthalmol 1984; 97:760–766.

Benedetto DA, Clinch TE, Laibson PR. In vivo observation of tear dynamics using fluorophotometry. Arch Ophthalmol 1984;102:410–412.

Birren JE, Casperson RC, Botwinick J. Age changes in pupil size. J Gerontol 1950; 5:267–271.

Cooper BA, Ward MW, Gowland CA, McIntosh JM. The use of the lanthony new color test in determining the effects of aging on color vision. J Gerontol 1991;46(6):320–324.

de Roetth A. Lacrimation in normal eyes. Arch Ophthalmol 1953;49:185–189.

Devaney KO, Johnson HA. Neuron loss in the aging visual cortex of man. J Gerontol 1980;35:836–841.

Dohlman CH. Physiology. *In* Smolin G, Thoft R (eds): The Cornea—Scientific Foundations and Clinical Practice. Boston, Little, Brown, 1983, pp. 3–17.

Domey RG, McFarland RA, Chadwick E. Threshold and rate of dark adaptation as functions of age and time. Hum Factors 1960; Aug:109–120.

Dorey CK, Wu G, Ebenstein D et al. Cell loss in the aging retina. Invest Ophthalmol Vis Sci 1989; 30(8):1691–1699.

Eisner A, Fleming SA, Klein M, Mouldin M. Sensitivities in older eyes with good acuity: Cross-sectional norms. Invest Ophthalmol Vis Sci 1987; 28:1824–1831.

Elliott DB. Contrast Sensitivity with Aging: A Neural or Optical Phenomenon? Ophthalmic Physiol Opt 1987;7:415–419.

Elliott D, Whitaker D, Macveigh D. Neural contribution to spatiotemporal contrast sensitivity decline in healthy aging eyes. Vision Res 1990;30:541–547.

Exford J. A longitudinal study of refractive trends after age forty. Am J Optom Arch Am Acad Optom 1965; 42:685–692.

Fisher RF. Presbyopia and the changes with age in the crystalline lens. J Physiol 1973; 228:765–779.

Gartner S, Henkind P. Aging and degeneration of the human macula. 1. Outer nuclear layer and photoreceptors. Br J Opthalmol 1981; 65:23–28.

Goldman JN, Benedek GB, Dohlman CH, Kravitt B. Structural alterations affecting transparency in swollen human corneas. Invest Ophthalmol 1968; 7(5):501–519.

Haas A, Flammer J, Schneider U. Influence of age on the visual fields of normal subjects. Am J Ophthalmol 1986; 101:199–203.

Hamano T, Mitsunaga S, Kotani S, et al. Tear volume in relation to contact lens wear and age. Contact Lens Association of Ophthalmologists 1990; 16(1):57–61.

Henderson JW, Prough WA. Influence of age and sex on flow of tears. Arch Ophthalmol 1950; 43:224–231.

Hirsch MJ. Changes in astigmatism after forty. Am J Optom 1959; 36:395–405.

Jaffe GJ, Alvarado JA, Juster RP. Age-related changes of the normal visual field. Arch Ophthamol 1986; 104:1021–1025.

Jay JL, Mammo RB, Allan D. Effect of age on visual acuity after cataract extraction. Br J Ophthalmol 1987; 71:112–115.

Johnson CA, Adams AJ, Twelker JD, Quigg JM. Age-related changes in the central visual field for short-wavelength sensitive pathways. J Opt Soc Am 1988; 5:2131–9.

Katz J, Sommer A. A longitudinal study of the age-adjusted variability of automated visual fields. Arch Ophthalmol 1987; 105:1083–1086.

Kline DW, Schieber F. Vision and aging. *In* Birren JE, Schaie KW (eds): Handbook of the Psychology of Aging. New York, Van Nostrand Reinhold, 1985, pp. 296–331.

Klyce SD, Beuerman RW. Structure and function of the cornea. *In* Kaufman HE, Barron BA, McDonald MB, Waltman SR (eds): The Cornea. New York, Churchill Livingston, 1988, pp. 3–54.

Knoblauch K, Saunders F, Kusuda M et al. Age and illuminance effects in the Farnsworth-Munsell 100 hue test. Applied Optics 1987; 26(8):1441–1448.

Lavery JR, Gibson JM, Shaw DE, Rosenthal AR. Refraction and refractive errors in an elderly population. Ophthalmic Physiol Opt 1988; 8:394–396.

Lerman S. An experimental and clinical evaluation of lens transparency and aging. J Gerontol 1983; 38(3):293–301.

Loewenfeld IE. Pupillary changes related to age. *In* Thompson HS, Daroff R, Frisen L et al. (eds): Topics in Neuro-Ophthalmology. Baltimore, Williams and Wilkins, 1979, pp. 124–150.

Lynn JR, Fellman RL, Starita RJ. Exploring the normal visual field. *In* Ritch R, Shields MB, Krupin T (eds): The Glaucomas. St. Louis, C.V. Mosby, 1989, pp. 361–392.

Marmor MF. Visual changes with age. *In* Caird FI, Williamson J (eds): The Eye and Its Disorders in the Elderly. Bristol, Scotland, Wright. 1986, pp. 28–36.

Marshall J, Grindle J, Ansell PL, Borwein B. Convolution in human rods: An aging process. Br J Ophthalmol 1979; 63:181–187.

Mellerio J. Light absorption and scatter in the human lens. Vision Res 1971; 11:129–141.

Mellerio J. Yellowing of the human lens: Nuclear and cortical contributions. Vision Res 1987; 27(9):1581–1587.

Milder B. The lacrimal apparatus. *In* Moses RA, Hart WM (eds): Adlers Physiology of the Eye. St. Louis, C.V. Mosby 1987, p. 5.

Millodot M, O'Leary D. The Discrepancy between retinoscopic and subjective measurements: Effect of age. American Journal of Optometry and Physiological Optics 1978; 55(5):309–316.

Morgan MW. Changes in visual function in the aging eye. *In* Rosenbloom AA, Morgan MW (eds): Vision and Aging. New York, Fairchild, 1986, pp. 121–134.

Morrison JD, McGrath C. Assessment of the optical contributions to the age-related deterioration in vision. QJ Exp Physiol 1985; 70:249–269.

Moses RA. Accommodation. *In* Moses RA, Hart WM (eds): Adlers Physiology of the Eye. St. Louis, C.V. Mosby, 1987, pp. 291–310.

Moses RA. The eyelids. *In* Moses RA, Hart WM (eds): Adlers Physiology of the Eye. St. Louis, C.V. Mosby, 1987, pp. 1–14.

Owsley C, Gardner T, Sekuler R, Lieberman H. Role of the crystalline lens in the spatial vision loss of the elderly. Invest Ophthalmol Vis Sci 1985; 26:1165–1170.

Paschides CA, Petroutsos G, Psilas K. Correlation of conjunctival impression cytology with lacrimal function and age. Acta Ophthalmol (Copenh) 1991; 69 (4):422–425.

Patel S, Farrell JC. Age-related changes in precorneal tear film stability. Optom Vis Sci 1989; 66:175.

Pitts DG. The effects of aging on selected visual functions: Dark adaptation, visual acuity, stereopsis, and brightness contrast. *In* Sekuler R, Kline D, Dismukes K (eds): Aging and Human Visual Function. New York, Alan R. Liss, 1982.

Pokorny J, Smith V, Lutze M. Aging of the human lens. Applied Optics 1987; 26(8):1437–1440.

Repka MX, Quigley HA. The effect of age on normal human optic nerve fiber number and diameter. Ophthalmology 1989; 96(1):26–31.

Robertson GW, Yudkin J. Effect of age on dark adaptation. J Physiol 1944; 103:1–8.

Roy MS, Podgor MJ, Collier B, Gunkel RD. Color vision and age in a normal North American population. Graefe's Archive for clinical and experimental Ophthalmology 1991; 229:139–144.

Saunders H. Changes in the axis of astigmatism: A longitudinal study. Ophthalmic Physiol Opt 1988; 8:37–42.

Scheibel ME, Lindsay RD, Tomiyasu U, Scheibel AB. Progressive dendritic changes in aging human cortex. Exp Neurol 1975; 47:392–403.

Slataper FJ. Age norms of refraction and vision. Arch Ophthalmol 1950; 43(3):466–481.

Tripathi RC, Tripathi BJ. Lens morphology, aging, and cataract. J Gerontol 1983; 38(3):258–270.

Tsai CS, Ritch R, Shin DH et al. Age-related decline of disc rim area in visually normal subjects. Ophthalmology 1992; 99:29–35.

Verriest G. Further studies on acquired deficiency of color discrimination. J Opt Soc Am 1963; 53:185–95.

Verriest G, Laethem JV, Uvijls A. A new assessment of the normal ranges of the Farnsworth-Munsell 100 Hue Test scores. Am J Ophthalmol 1982; 93:635–642.

Waring GO, Bourne WM, Edelhauser HF, Kenyon KR. The corneal endothelium. Ophthalmol 1981; 89:531–590.

Weale RA. Age and the transmittance of the human crystalline lens. J Physiol 1988; 395:577–587.

Weale RA. Senile changes in visual acuity. Trans Ophthal Soc U.K. 1975; 95:36–38.

Weale RA. Spatial and temporal resolution. *In* The Aging Eye. New York, Harper and Row, 1963, pp. 144–153.

Werner EB. Manual of Visual Fields. New York, Churchill Livingstone, 1991, pp. 91–110.

Werner JS. Steele VG. Sensitivity of human foveal color mechanisms throughout the life span. J Opt Soc Am [A] 1988; 5:2122–2130.

Werner JS, Peterzell DH, Scheetz AJ. Light, vision, and aging. Optom Vis Sci 1990; 67:214–229.

Wright CE, Drasdo N. The influence on the spatial and temporal contrast sensitivity function. Doc. Ophthalmology 1985; 59:385–395.

Zigman S. Ultra violet light and human lens pigmentation. Vision Res 1978; 18:509–514.

6

Geriatric Ocular Disease

Timothy Harkins

This chapter reviews the typical clinical characteristics and management of frequently encountered geriatric ocular diseases. Because most eye diseases are seen with greater frequency with advancing age, most eye diseases will be given consideration, but the reader is reminded that a comprehensive review is not possible in a single chapter. For more complete information, please refer to the citations provided at the end of the chapter.

DIAGNOSTIC PRINCIPLES

Proper diagnosis requires effective problem-solving strategies. Early hypothesis formation and constant hypothesis refinement is a useful approach (Kelly, 1989). This technique involves developing a list of hypothetical diagnoses (differential diagnosis) at the outset of the examination. Tests are then chosen to support or refute the possibilities. Test results are interpreted to refine and rank the list, and additional tests can be used for confirmation.

Each piece of subjective or objective data can be used in this technique. From the outset, a patient's age, race, and gender provide demographic data that help form or rank a diagnostic list (e.g., cataracts increase in frequency with age, glaucoma is more common in blacks, and Fuchs' dystrophy is more common in women). The patient's symptoms provide a starting point for choosing tests (burning eyes are more likely anterior segment disease, while decreased visual acuity mandates evaluation of refractive error, media, macula, and optic nerve). Test results then restructure the list of hypotheticals (refraction may resolve decreased acuity, whereas an afferent pupillary defect implicates the optic nerve or a large retinal lesion). Further tests based on preliminary findings are chosen to confirm the hypothesis (the afferent pupillary defect compels evaluation of the optic nerve and the likely causes of optic neuropathy).

Employing this strategy has some requirements. Optometrists must know the relative frequency of diseases, the manifestations of diseases, the tests that will yield these manifestations, and how to perform and interpret these tests.

Making a diagnosis is easier when the diagnosis is anticipated (based on an early hypothesis), although care must be taken to avoid biasing test results.

It is helpful to remember that there are four broad types of findings. In order of frequency they are typical manifestations of common diseases, atypical manifestations of common diseases, typical manifestations of uncommon diseases, and atypical manifestations of uncommon diseases.

Finally, it is important to note that a diagnosis is not an end—the patient's problems must still be resolved. Management decisions are not based solely on the diagnosis but also on the patient's complaints, the prognosis, and on the risk-benefit ratio of therapy.

THE EYELIDS
Inflammation

Blepharitis Blepharitis is a common cause of eyelid inflammation and external eye irritation. Staphylococcus colonization is frequently the cause. Patients can present with complaints of burning, itching, dry eye, and epiphora. The typical clinical sign is a collarette surrounding individual lashes. Other clinical signs include missing or misdirected lashes and inflamed or ulcerated lid margins. Blepharitis is often the cause of hordeola and chalazia. The tear film can be less full and less clean, resulting in dry eye signs and symptoms. Inferior corneal epitheliopathy can also result from blepharitis (McCulley, 1983).

There is no cure for blepharitis, but the problem can be controlled with chronic treatment. The therapy depends on the severity of the signs and symptoms, as well as on the patient's ability to participate in self-care. Conservative management is centered around improved hygiene to reduce the colonization of bacteria. Gentle lid scrubs with warm water (taking care not to be too abrasive to an already compromised lid margin) can be done nightly or twice daily. Lid scrubs with diluted baby shampoo can be more effective, but this is often toxic to the lids, too cumbersome to expect chronic compliance, and frequently misunderstood as "baby oil" scrubs. Bacitracin ointment (alternatively erythromycin) is the antibiotic of choice because of its specific anti-gram positive activity and is used in severe cases or when compliance with lid scrubs cannot be expected. If there is an associated dry eye, it should be treated also (McCulley, 1984).

Meibomianitis Meibomianitis is commonly seen with blepharitis and the symptoms are similar. Because the meibomian glands play an important role in the development of the tear film, meibomianitis should be considered when dry eye cases are evaluated. Patients with meibomianitis often have rosacea. This diagnosis can be made by looking for the facial characteristics of rosacea, which are flushing, erythema, telangiectasia, papules, pustules, and rhinophyma (Griffith, 1987). Clinical signs depend on the degree of altered meibomian secretions. They range from foamy, impure secretions to inspissated secretions to completely plugged orifices. The secretions are evaluated by digitally forcing them from the gland (Catania, 1988).

Meibomianitis is treated either conservatively or aggressively. It is conservatively managed with warm compresses (to dilate the orifices), followed by gently massaging secretions from the glands. Aggressive management is with tetracycline, which is often indicated when there is associated rosacea. As with blepharitis, it is important to treat a concurrent dry eye.

Structural Anomalies

Entropion Entropion in the elderly is either involutional or cicatricial. Both result in trichiasis, and patients will complain of chronically irritated eyes; their corneas may be at risk for mechanical abrasion. Surgery is the required treatment.

Ectropion Ectropion in the elderly is usually involutional but can be cicatricial or paralytic (cranial nerve VII palsy). Epiphora can result because tears do not have access to the lower puncta. More seriously, dry eye can result because of poor distribution and exposure. Lubricants are indicated until the ectropion resolves or until surgery corrects the problem.

Blepharoptosis Acquired blepharoptosis can be neurologic (Horner's and myasthenia gravis should be considered) or traumatic but usually results from dermatochalasis. Evaluation includes measuring the vertical palpebral fissure, the distance from the upper lid margin to the pupillary reflex, and the upper lid's range of motion. Visual field with the lid untaped and taped will document the effect of the ptosis on vision and the potential improvement after surgical correction. Symptoms and degree of visual dysfunction will dictate whether surgery is indicated (Katowitz, 1990).

Neoplasms

In evaluating eyelid neoplasms, the practitioner must make one critical decision, whether the lesion is malignant or benign. The most common malignancies of the lids are basal cell carcinoma and squamous cell carcinoma (Griffith, 1987).

Malignant Neoplasms

Basal cell carcinomas make up nearly 90% of eyelid malignancies. Long-term ultraviolet (UV) exposure is a causative risk factor, and fair-skinned people are at highest risk. The lower eyelid and medial canthus are the most likely sites for basal cell lesions. They are seen less frequently on the upper lid because of the protection of the brow. The classic description of basal cell carcinoma is a lesion with firm, raised, pearly nodules with or without telangectasia and an ulcerated center (Figure 6-1). Prompt surgical removal is indicated.

Squamous cell carcinoma manifests as a flesh colored nodule of keratin with an ulcerated center (often covered with scales) on sun-damaged skin. It is less

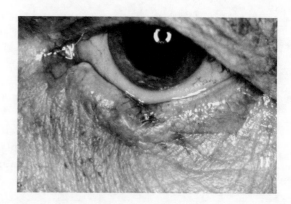

Figure 6-1 Basal cell carcinoma (courtesy of Tom Lutz, O.D.).

common than basal cell but more aggressive in nature. As with basal cell carcinoma, prompt surgical removal is indicated.

Benign Neoplasms

Benign lid lesions in the elderly include xanthalasma (Figure 6-2), papilloma (Figure 6-3), epidermal inclusion cysts, seborrheic keratosis, and actinic keratosis. They can be removed for cosmetic reasons.

THE TEAR FILM
Dry Eye

The tear film has a variety of roles in maintaining corneal integrity—lubrication, disinfection, and removal of debris. A reduced tear film will result in dry eye symptoms of burning, scratching, redness, and excessive lacrimation. There are many tests for evaluating the status of the tear film, but usually clinical signs can be found to correlate with symptoms without performing an elaborate workup. The height of the lacrimal lake, the amount of debris in the tears, and the

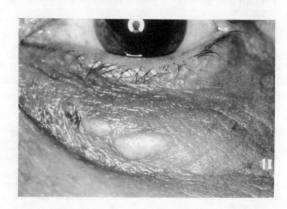

Figure 6-2 Xanthalasma (courtesy of Tom Lutz, O.D.).

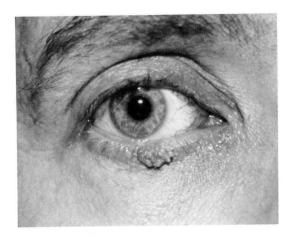

Figure 6-3 Papilloma (courtesy of Tom Lutz, O.D.).

tear break-up time can be observed readily and compared with those in patients without symptoms. The inferior corneal epithelium can be compromised in severe cases; fluorescein or rose bengal staining make this observation more apparent. Commonly associated conditions such as blepharitis, meibomianitis, lagophthalmos, and ectropion should be considered because their presence may alter management decisions.

There are many treatment options. Underlying causes should be identified and treated. When associated blepharitis and meibomianitis are controlled, the dry eye symptoms will be reduced. Ectropion repair should be considered. Lagophthalmos dictates more aggressive management during sleep. Primary therapy for dry eye is tear supplementation—drops as needed during the day and ointment at bedtime. Nonpreserved tear supplements should be used if a reaction to the preservatives is suspected. Some patients benefit from punctal occlusion to slow tear outflow. Permanent occlusion (either with plugs or cicatrization) should always be preceded by a trial with temporary collagen plugs to reduce the risk of iatrogenic epiphora.

Outflow Disorders

Tear outflow disorders will result in epiphora. Diagnosis begins by ruling out causes of excessive lacrimation (dry eye, infection). Observation of a puncta not in close apposition to the globe is diagnostic. Diagnosis can also be made by observing asymmetric clearance of dye from the tear film or failure of dye to drain to the nose or back of the throat (Jones test). Lacrimal probing and irrigation can identify and occasionally clear obstruction in the upper lacrimal system. This should never be done when infection is the suspected cause of obstruction. When irrigation is unsuccessful or in lower lacrimal system disorders, surgery is indicated (Katowitz, 1990).

CORNEA
Dystrophies

Epithelial Basement Membrane Dystrophy   Epithelial basement membrane dystrophy can manifest itself in the pattern of maps, dots, and fingerprints, or in combinations of these patterns. Most patients are asymptomatic, but recurrent epithelial erosions can occur. Symptoms are similar to symptoms with any abrasion but are usually noted upon waking and without a history of trauma. Initial treatment is to heal the abrasion and prevent infection. Once completely healed, prophylactic use of lubricant or hypertonic ointment is prescribed.

Fuchs' Endothelial Dystrophy   Fuchs' endothelial dystrophy is most often seen in the elderly, with a higher frequency in women than in men. It begins with endothelial compromise, manifested clinically as guttata and a reduction in the number of endothelial cells. Because the compromised endothelium is a less efficient pump, stromal edema results. Stromal edema rarely causes reduced vision but will if the corneal thickness is significant (>0.65mm). Epithelial edema results when the endothelial pump is not efficient enough to eliminate fluid from the cornea at the eye's specific intraocular pressure, that is, epithelial edema is dependent on endothelial function and intraocular pressure (IOP). Epithelial edema does cause reduced vision and is the most common cause of symptoms in patients with Fuchs'. Therapy is aimed at reducing the epithelial edema by use of hypertonic solutions and ointment. Ocular hypotensive drops may help. Penetrating keratoplasy is the definitive treatment.

Degenerations

Pterygia are fibrovascular growth of conjunctiva onto the corneal epithelium (Figure 6-4). They are usually in the nasal palpebral fissure and grow centrally from the limbus. Pterygia are seen more frequently in people who have spent more time outdoors because UV exposure, dry heat, and wind are suspected to

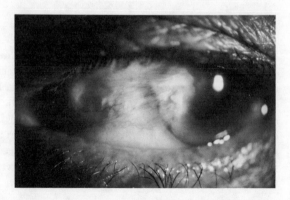

Figure 6-4   Pterygium (photo Jeff Ellenwood).

play a role in their development. Many pterygia do not affect vision, but the likelihood increases as the pterygia advances toward the center. Visual compromise begins with refractive error change (increasing with the rule and irregular astigmatism) and worsens as the ptergium crosses the visual axis. Progression can be monitored by measuring the pterygium with the slit beam in the biomicroscope or with photography. Treatment is surgical removal, although recurrences are common (Arffa, 1991).

THE LENS
Cataracts

Nuclear sclerotic cataracts make the lens appear hazy gray and often yellow or brown. They can cause refractive error shifts (usually toward myopia), decreased visual acuity, decreased contrast sensitivity, and increased sensitivity to glare. Cortical changes appear as spokelike opacities, usually beginning peripherally and progressing to the center of the lens. Cortical spokes are more frequently associated with glare than with decreased visual acuity. Posterior subcapsular cataracts are dense, central, posterior opacities seen in a wide range of sizes. They result in decreased visual acuity that is more marked when the pupil is small.

Cataract evaluation begins with a history, specifically to determine whether the patient is experiencing decreased vision and under what circumstances. After refraction, the patient's symptoms may be observed clinically by measuring visual acuity in dark and normal room illumination, acuity in the presence of glare, reading acuity, or by measuring contrast sensitivity. The lens should be examined to correlate its appearance with the patient's symptoms and visual function status. Other causes of decreased vision should be ruled out.

Cataract surgery is elective and the decision to perform surgery is based on the patient's desire to improve vision and the doctor's expectations for improved vision after surgery.

Pseudophakia

Cataract surgery has a high success rate and a low complication rate. Most patients are left pseudophakic with a posterior chamber implant. These lenses create few complications. Because an intact posterior capsule is required, posterior chamber lenses are associated with (but do not cause) posterior capsular fibrosis. This fibrosis occurs in roughly one third of posterior chamber implant patients as a result of proliferation of anterior capsule cells across the surface of the posterior capsule. When the fibrosis is central, vision is affected. Treatment is a capsulotomy with Nd:YAG laser.

Fewer cataract patients are left pseudophakic with an anterior chamber lens. These lenses are associated with a higher complication rate. Inflammation resulting from direct contact to the iris is not uncommon and can lead to cystoid macular edema. Treatment is with topical anti-inflammatory agents and cycloplegics. Corneal edema can result from the endothelial compromise caused by the direct trauma of an anterior chamber lens. This is treated with hyperosmotics and ocular hypotensives, although bullous keratopathy frequently develops and surgery is required. Damage to the trabecular meshwork (sometimes apparent gonioscopically) and anterior segment inflammation can cause increased IOP with anterior chamber lenses. Treatment is with ocular hypotensives.

Aphakia

Aphakia is a rare result of cataract extraction. Spectacles and contact lenses are used to correct the large refractive error. Cystoid macular edema, usually associated with anterior segment inflammation, can occur. Aphakic bullous keratopathy can result from endothelial compromise due to surgical trauma or vitreous touch. Peripheral vitreoretinal disease is more likely to advance to retinal detachment in the phakic eye than in phakic or pseudophakic eye.

THE RETINA
Vascular Retinal Disease

Diabetic Retinopathy Diabetic retinopathy is the most common cause of blindness in America. It is the retina's unique metabolic activity and vascularity that put it at risk for diabetic microvascular complications. Diabetic retinopathy can cause vision loss in either of two ways: reduced visual acuity resulting from diabetic maculopathy or profound vision loss resulting from proliferative retinopathy.

There are many classification systems for diabetic retinopathy, but it is most simply separated into three stages: background, preproliferative, and proliferative diabetic retinopathy. In background diabetic retinopathy, there are direct manifestations of microvasculopathy: hemorrhages, microaneurysms, and hard exudates. The important observation marking the advance to preproliferative retinopathy is ischemia (seen as cotton-wool spots), usually seen in addition to background findings. Other changes in preproliferative retinopathy are intraretinal microvascular abnormalities (IRMA) and venous beading. Proliferative disease is manifested as neovascularization.

Diabetic maculopathy can threaten vision in any of the three stages of retinopathy. It usually results from macular edema (caused by leaking microaneurysms near the macula), but can be caused by hypoxia (which is not treatable). The hallmark of macular edema is retinal thickening, which can be seen with or without hard exudates (Figure 6-5). Diabetic macular edema is often a treatable condition. Guidelines for when the risk-benefit ratio favors treatment of macular edema have been outlined by the Early Treatment for Diabetic Retinopathy Study Group (ETDRS) (1991). The ETDRS describes treatable clinically significant macular edema (CSME) in the following way: Retinal thickening at or within 500 μm of the center of the macula and/or hard exudates at or within 500 μm

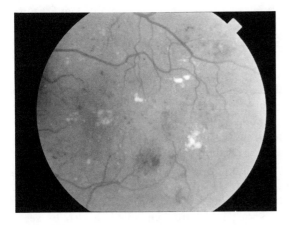

Figure 6-5 Clinically significant macular edema (courtesy of Jeff Ellenwood).

of the center of the macula, if associated with thickening of the adjacent retina; and/or a zone or zones of retinal thickening one disc area in size at least part of which was within one disc diameter of the center. Treatment is with focal photocoagulation; fluorescein angiography is required to guide treatment.

Proliferative disease is seen as neovascularization of the disc (NVD, Figure 6-6), neovascularization elsewhere (NVE), or neovascularization of the iris (rubeosis iridis). Proliferation can lead to three vision-threatening conditions: vitreous hemorrhage, traction retinal detachment, or neovascular glaucoma. The Diabetic Retinopathy Study Group (1981) has provided guidelines for the treatment of proliferative retinopathy: (1) NVD greater than one quarter the disc area, (2) NVD and preretinal or vitreous hemorrhage, and (3) NVE and preretinal or vitreous hemorrhage. Treatment is with scatter or pan-retinal photocoagulation

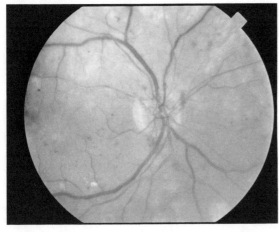

Figure 6-6 Neovascularization of the disc (courtesy of Jeff Ellenwood).

(PRP). More advanced complications of proliferative retinopathy may require vitrectomy. Neovascularization of the iris requires aggressive, usually complete, PRP. If glaucoma develops, aggressive ocular hypotensive therapy is required to prevent blindness and pain.

Vein Occlusions   After diabetic retinopathy, retinal vein occlusions are the second most common retinal vascular diseases seen. They can be classified as branch and central retinal vein occlusions. Systemic disease is frequently implicated in the development of vein occlusions; systemic hypertension, diabetes, hyperlipid-emias, and coagulopathies should be considered.

Branch vein occlusions are diagnosed ophthalmoscopically. Findings are tortuous and dilated veins with hemorrhages (dot, blot, and flame-shaped) that originate at the site of obstruction and radiate toward the periphery (Figure 6-7). Microaneurysms, cotton-wool spots, and hard exudates can also be seen. Findings are limited to a single quadrant (most commonly the superior temporal). Collateral vessels develop to improve impaired vascular drainage and can be confused with neovascularization. In most cases, it is possible to distinguish collaterals from neovascularization with ophthalmoscopic observation (without fluorescein angiography) by noting whether the vessels begin and end on a vein and whether they cross the retina's horizontal midline.

Branch vein occlusions can threaten vision in three ways: macular hypoxia, macular edema, and vitreous hemorrhage associated with neovascularization. Macular hypoxia is not treatable. The Branch Vein Occlusion Study Group (BVOS, 1984; BVOS, 1986) outlines treatment criteria to reduce vision loss from edema and vitreous hemorrhage. Macular edema present for 3 to 18 months, resulting in visual acuity 20/40 or worse, benefits from focal photocoagulation. Scatter photocoagulation to reduce the risk of vision loss from vitreous hemorrhage is recommended for branch vein occlusion only after the development of neovascu-larization.

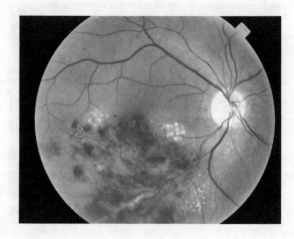

Figure 6-7 Branch retinal vein occlusion (courtesy of Jeff Ellenwood).

Patients with central retinal vein occlusion present with tortuous and dilated veins and hemorrhages in all four quadrants (Figure 6-8). As with branch vein occlusion (BRVO), systemic disease must be considered. Unlike BRVO, there is a strong correlation with underlying glaucoma in the affected or contralateral eye, and this must be evaluated as well. Vision can be threatened in either of two ways: Neovascular glaucoma (which rarely develops in branch vein occlusions) or maculopathy.

There are two different types of central retinal vein occlusion, but they have been described in many different ways. Because the development of iris neovascularization is strongly associated with the degree of retinal nonperfusion, the terms *perfused* and *nonperfused* are probably best. The Central Vein Occlusion Study (CVOS) has been designed to determine if prophylactic scatter photocoagulation is of benefit in preventing the development of neovascular glaucoma, but the study has not been completed. It is theorized that the larger the area of nonperfused retina, the greater the chance of neovascular glaucoma and the greater benefit from prophylaxis.

Persistent macular edema is a common cause of vision loss in central vein occlusion. The CVOS has been designed to determine the natural course and treatment guidelines for macular edema in central retinal vein occlusion; however, because the causes and manifestations appear similar to macular edema in branch retinal vein occlusion and diabetic retinopathy, the indications for treatment might be the same.

Artery Occlusions   Retinal arterial obstruction can be divided into central and branch retinal occlusions. Emboli are responsible for most retinal artery obstructions; less frequently the cause can be vasculitis, coagulopathies, trauma, or optic neuropathy. Common associated medical conditions are hypertension, cardiac disease, carotid stenosis, diabetes, and cholesterol abnormalities. The life

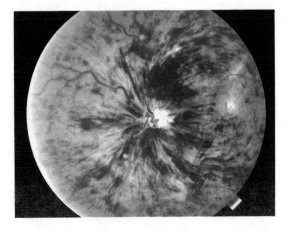

Figure 6-8   Central retinal vein occlusion (courtesy of Jeff Ellenwood).

expectancy of patients with retinal artery occlusions is reduced, and the most frequent causes of death are cardiovascular disease and stroke. Patients should be referred for a medical evaluation with a reminder to the physician of the common medical conditions and a suggestion to evaluate the patient's risk for heart attack or stroke (Alexander, 1992). Because giant cell arteritis can cause a central retinal artery occlusion (although rarely) and because this can quickly lead to blindness in the other eye, a stat Westergren's sedimentation rate should be ordered to rule out this possible cause.

Central retinal artery occlusions present with symptoms of acute loss of vision. There is an afferent pupillary defect, and the retina appears opacified, with the exception of the macula, where a cherry red spot is seen. The arteries can appear attenuated. The emboli may or may not be present on examination. After several weeks, the retina will often appear normal with the exception of thinned arteries and optic nerve atrophy. Therapy is effective only if started within hours of vision loss, and then prognosis remains poor. Anterior chamber paracentesis, ocular massage, hyperventilation, and oxygen–carbon dioxide mixture have been suggested for therapy.

Branch artery occlusion findings are similar to those in central retinal artery occlusion but are limited to a single quadrant, and visual acuity might be spared (Figure 6-9). Prognosis is quite good; about 80% resolve with 20/40 vision or better. There is no ocular treatment, although systemic diagnosis and management is critical. Referral for medical care is the same as for central retinal artery occlusion (Ryan, 1989).

Macular Disease

Age-related Macular Degeneration Age-related macular degeneration (ARMD) is a leading cause of reduced functional vision in the geriatric population. The critical decision to be made when a patient with ARMD is evaluated is

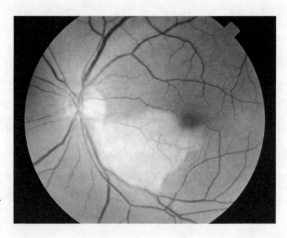

Figure 6-9 Branch retinal artery occlusion (courtesy of Jeff Ellenwood).

whether there is associated choroidal neovascularization (CNV). This decision is necessary because CNV can be treatable, whereas other changes in ARMD are degenerative and not treatable.

Atrophic changes seen in ARMD are drusen (soft, hard, or mixed); retinal pigment epithelium hyper- or hypopigmentation, and areas of geographic atrophy. There is associated visual acuity loss, usually not beyond 20/200. There is no treatment to reverse or halt the atrophy.

The atrophic changes of ARMD predispose the eye for the development of CNV. The important symptom associated with CNV is that straight lines appear distorted or wavy. Patients can see this when they look at an Amsler grid or may notice it on any line that they know should appear straight. Hemorrhage, elevation, and exudate are the biomicroscopic (with auxiliary lens) findings that are suggestive of CNV (Figure 6-10). Hemorrhage can be seen as red (hemorrhage internal to the pigment epithelium) or dirty gray-green (hemorrhage posterior to and discolored by the pigment epithelium). Elevation can be best appreciated with stereopsis and is the manifestation of leaking CNV. Hard exudates are rarely seen without other indicators of CNV and are another manifestation of leakage. Success of treatment with focal laser photocoagulation is dependent on location of the neovascular membrane (located with fluorescein angiography) and extent of present damage (Bressler, 1988).

Internal Limiting Membrane Retinopathy Internal limiting membrane (ILM) retinopathy can cause symptomatic visual acuity loss when the macula is involved. ILM retinopathy is caused by a migration of glial cells through a dehiscence in the ILM after a posterior vitreous detachment. These cells proliferate across the ILM, distorting the retinal surface. Therapy to improve visual acuity is with vitrectomy and membrane peel—a complicated, invasive technique with a risk to benefit ratio that favors treatment only when acuity is markedly reduced (Ryan, 1989).

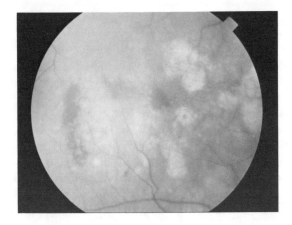

Figure 6-10 Age-related macular degeneration with hemorrhage suggestive of choroidal neovascularization (courtesy of Jeff Ellenwood).

Macular Holes Macular holes are a result of posterior vitreous detachments with enough retinal adhesion to detach the superficial layers of the retina along with the vitreous. There is no treatment to replace the detached macular layers. Bilateral retinal holes occur approximately 25% of the time. Upon diagnosis of a unilateral macular hole, the other eye should be carefully evaluated for vitreous traction at the macula, and prophylactic vitrectomy should be considered cautiously (Gass, 1989).

Peripheral Retinal Disease

Retinal Breaks Lesions predisposing to retinal detachment are seen more frequently with increasing age. Atrophic holes rarely progress to clinical retinal detachment and are seldom treated prophylactically. The natural history of untreated lattice degeneration is that it progresses to clinical retinal detachment in only 1% of eyes over 10 years, and prophylaxis is rarely indicated (Byer, 1989). Asymptomatic retinal tears in phakic, nonfellow eyes (i.e., where the fellow eye does not have a history of detachment) do not progress to detachment often enough to justify unconditional prophylaxis (Byer, 1982). Retinal tears in which prophylaxis is warranted (because of their increased likelihood to lead to detachment) are those with symptoms (most important indicator), in aphakia (or pseudophakia), in fellow eyes, and in eyes on cholinergic therapy. Prophylactic treatment is with photocoagulation or cryotherapy.

Retinal Detachment Retinal detachment is seen as serous elevation (best seen with indirect ophthalmoscopy) of all or part of the sensory retina. Careful observation will usually reveal the causal retinal break. Treatment is to restore apposition of the sensory retina to the pigment epithelium (with scleral buckle or pneumatic retinopexy) and to close the retinal break, usually with cryotherapy (Schepens, 1983).

THE OPTIC NERVE
The Glaucomas

The glaucomas are a group of diseases whose common denominator is optic neuropathy; they are the most common causes of optic atrophy. Most glaucomas are associated with increased IOP, but IOP is not considered a very sensitive or specific diagnostic tool because many patients with glaucoma have statistically normal IOP, and conversely, many healthy patients have statistically high IOP. Diagnosis is made by careful stereoscopic observation of the optic nerve head, looking for characteristic glaucomatous excavation. Retinal nerve fiber layer defects may heighten suspicion for glaucomatous damage. The presence of characteristic glaucomatous optic atrophy prompts visual field testing to evaluate functional status of the optic nerve. Characteristic visual field changes in glaucoma are nasal steps, paracentral scotomas, arcuate defects, and generalized reduced sensitivity.

Visual field loss should always be interpreted in light of optic nerve and nerve fiber layer appearances.

Types of Glaucoma

The optic nerve's physical characteristics and functional status will determine the presence or absence of glaucoma. IOP, anterior segment evaluation and gonioscopy are used to diagnose the type of glaucoma, for example, open angle or closed angle, primary or secondary glaucoma.

Primary Open Angle Glaucoma   Primary open angle glaucoma (POAG) is the most frequently diagnosed glaucoma. These patients have normal gonioscopic and anterior segment findings and their IOP is beyond statistically normal.

Low Tension Glaucoma   Low tension glaucoma (LTG) has findings similar to POAG except that multiple examinations fail to yield increased IOP.

Secondary Glaucomas   Secondary glaucomas may be diagnosed by observing anterior segment inflammation, trabecular meshwork hyperpigmentation, pseudoexfoliation material, or rubeosis.

Angle Closure Glaucoma   Acute angle closure glaucoma is rare. Typical clinical signs are corneal edema, very high IOP, a mid-dilated pupil, and a gonioscopically occluded angle. Subacute angle closure glaucoma is not rare and is the most misdiagnosed of all glaucomas. Patients do not have acutely elevated IOP but have a gonioscopically occludable angle (with peripheral anterior synechia indicating previous occlusion).

Glaucoma Therapy

POAG   There are a variety of therapies for primary open angle glaucoma with a wide range of efficacy and a wide range of potential adverse effects. The goal is to lower the IOP to a safe level at which there is no longer advance of the optic atrophy or visual field. From conservative to aggressive the therapies include topical ocular hypotensive agents (beta blockers, cholinergics, and adrenergics); systemic carbonic anhydrase inhibitors; argon laser trabeculoplasty (ALT); and filtering surgery.

Secondary Glaucomas   Secondary glaucomas have similar therapies, with reduced options depending on the primary cause. Cholinergics and adrenergics are contraindicated in inflammatory glaucoma, and ALT and filtering procedures are less effective in inflammatory glaucoma. Pilocarpine and ALT can be more effective in pigmentary glaucoma, whereas ALT can be more effective in exfoliation glaucoma. Adrenergics and cholinergics are contraindicated in rubeotic glaucoma, whereas ALT is ineffective and filtering procedures less effective in rubeotic glaucoma.

Angle Closure Glaucoma Acute angle closure glaucoma requires prompt reduction of the IOP. Glycerin (osmoglyn) (about mL/lb) is used when not contraindicated by diabetes or congestive heart failure. If contraindicated by diabetes, it is replaced by isosorbide (1.5 mL/lb). The patient can be given two 250-mg tablets of acetazolamide (Diamox) and a drop of timolol (Timoptic). Intermittent dynamic gonioscopy is used to change the pressure dynamics of the anterior segment and move aqueous from posterior chamber to anterior chamber. Then the patient is made to lie on his or her back to help the lens move posteriorly. Pilocarpine is not used until the attack has been broken, because it moves the lens anteriorly, exacerbating the pupillary block. Once the attack is broken and IOP is controlled, laser peripheral iridotomy is performed.

Subacute angle closure is treated with laser peripheral iridotomy. Statistically, patients with angle closure are likely to have an open angle component of glaucoma as well (because of previous damage to the trabecular meshwork and the optic nerve); if present, this should be treated after the iridotomy (Epstein, 1986; Ritch, 1989; Shields, 1992).

Optic Nerve Edema

The inflamed or swollen optic nerve head is readily apparent on internal examination. With stereopsis, the nerve head is elevated, it is hyperemic, the venous pulse is absent, the associated nerve fiber layer is opaque, and there are often splinter hemorrhages and retinal edema (Figure 6-11). The initial decision should be whether one or both eyes are involved because this has an impact on the differential diagnosis and work-up.

Papilledema Bilateral disc edema is termed *papilledema* and is associated with elevated intracranial pressure. This should be considered medically emergent. Measure blood pressure because hypertension can be a cause and order radiologic

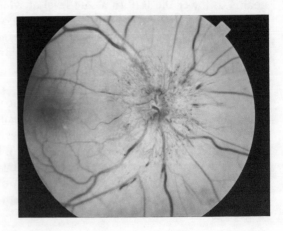

Figure 6-11 Optic nerve edema (courtesy off Jeff Ellenwood).

studies (to look for an intracranial mass). In the geriatric population, pseudotumor cerebri is unlikely (and is a diagnosis of exclusion in anyone).

Unilateral Disc Edema   Finding the cause of unilateral disc edema is more difficult. This should also be considered medically emergent because one of the causes—giant cell arteritis—can quickly cause blindness in the other eye. The causes can be divided most easily into four categories: vascular, inflammatory, compressive, or ocular.

Vascular causes of optic nerve edema are giant cell arteritis or nonarteritic ischemic optic neuropathy. Associated findings in giant cell arteritis are headache, malaise, weakness, weight loss, jaw pain, and polymyalagia. Order a Westergren sedimentation rate and complete blood count stat. A sufficiently elevated sedimentation rate suggests a preliminary diagnosis of giant cell arteritis, and high-dose steroids should be begun to reduce risk of blindness of the other eye (assuming the complete blood count indicated no acute infection). Temporal artery biopsy yields a more definite diagnosis.

Nonarteric ischemic optic neuropathy is a more likely diagnosis. It is theorized to be a result of atherosclerotic disease. Patients usually have small optic nerve heads and small cup-to-disc ratios. (This structure has been implicated as a cause of ischemic optic neuropathy.) Hypertension and diabetes are frequently associated findings and should be considered in the differential diagnosis, although a specific cause is often not found. Nonarteritic ischemic optic neuropathy can be progressive or nonprogressive. The progressive form might benefit from optic nerve sheath fenestration, but nonprogressive ischemic optic neuropathy is not treatable.

While not common, inflammatory causes should be considered in optic nerve edema. Clues to postviral syndrome come from a careful case history. Syphilis, collagen vascular diseases, sarcoidosis, and tuberculosis can be ruled out with carefully considered laboratory tests.

Radiology of the nerve and orbit is used to evaluate for compressive optic neuropathy. Thyroid orbitopathy and meningiomas are the most likely compressive causes in this population.

Vein occlusion, uveitis, and hypotony can cause optic nerve edema and are readily evaluated in the eye examination.

Optic Nerve Atrophy

Optic nerve atrophy can be manifested as pallor with or without excavation (Figure 6-12). The differential diagnosis is broader than optic nerve edema, because prolonged optic nerve edema can result in optic nerve atrophy, so the same causes must be considered: vascular, inflammatory, compressive, and ocular. Recall that glaucoma is the most common cause of optic atrophy and should always be considered regardless of IOP. Additionally considered are toxicity, nutritional deficiency, and trauma (Bajandas and Kline, 1988).

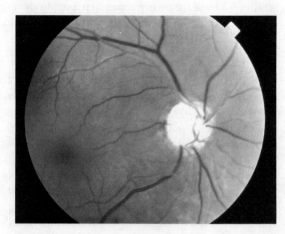

Figure 6-12 Syphilitic optic neuropathy mimicking glaucoma (courtesy of Jeff Ellenwood).

NEURO-OPHTHALMIC DISEASE
The Visual Field

The visual field can be affected by lesions anywhere along the visual pathway beginning at the retina and ending at the occipital lobe. Fortunately, each site has specific characteristics that often make localizing the lesion a straightforward task:

Retina
1. Defects do not respect the vertical or horizontal midline.
2. Visual acuity is reduced if the macula is involved.
3. Afferent pupil defect is present if lesion is large enough and monocular.
4. Defects may be bilateral but not congruous; asymmetry is the rule.
5. Diagnosis is by internal examination.

Optic Nerve
1. Does not respect vertical midline but can respect horizontal midline.
2. Visual acuity is reduced if temporal fibers are affected.
3. Afferent pupil defect is present if lesion is asymmetric.
4. Defects may be bilateral, but not congruous; asymmetry is the rule.
5. Visual field defects respect nerve fiber bundles: papillomacular bundle, arcuate nerve fiber bundle, and nasal nerve fiber bundle.

Optic Chiasm
1. Site of bitemporal field loss.
2. Not the site of binasal field loss; binasal defects are from bilateral retina or nerve lesions.
3. Defects may be asymmetric if chiasm and one nerve are involved (junctional lesion).

Post-Chiasm
1. Homonymous defects are the rule.
2. Congruity increases as lesions move posteriorly. Congruity only describes incomplete hemianopias; complete hemianopias cannot be localized.
3. Temporal lobe lesions are denser superiorly.
4. Parietal lobe lesions are denser inferiorly and are associated with optokinetic nystagmus asymmetry.
5. Visual acuity is unaffected unless bilateral lesions are present.
6. Tip of occipital lobe represents macular fibers. Lesions may affect this part of field in isolation or may spare this part of field.
7. Cerebrovascular accidents are the cause of 90% of homonymous hemianopias (Bajandas and Kline, 1988; Feldon, 1989).

Oculomotor Nerve Palsy

Oculomotor nerve (cranial nerve III) palsies may affect an isolated muscle, the pupil, cause ptosis, or combinations of these. Patients will complain of new-onset diplopia. There will be exotropia that increases with gaze toward the involved muscle. If the pupil is involved, this is a medical emergency, and a posterior communicating artery aneurysm must be ruled out as soon as possible. If the pupil is spared, microvasculopathy is the likely cause (consider postviral effects, diabetes, and hypertension), and the diplopia will resolve in about 3 months. If the palsy persists beyond 3 months, radiologic studies should be ordered to rule out a neoplasm.

Trochlear Nerve Palsy

New-onset vertical diplopia is nearly always a result of trochlear nerve palsy (cranial nerve IV) affecting the superior oblique muscle. This can be confirmed by the three-step test: The first step is to identify the eye with hyperdeviation. The deviation will increase with gaze to the opposite side (second step) and increase with head tilt to the same side (third step). Vascular causes (postviral effects, diabetes, and hypertension) and traumatic causes are most common. Vascular lesions will resolve in about 3 months. Palsies lasting beyond 3 months should be evaluated with radiology to rule out the rare compressive lesion.

Abducens Nerve Palsy

Abducens nerve palsy (cranial nerve VI) will result in esotropia that increases with gaze toward the involved muscle. Microvasculopathy (postviral effects, diabetes, and hypertension) is again the likely cause and resolution is again likely in 3 months. If the palsy persists beyond 3 months, radiology should be ordered to rule out a mass lesion.

Bell's Palsy

The other important cranial nerve palsy in geriatrics is Bell's palsy (cranial nerve VII). There is a characteristic facial droop, and the important complication in eye care is the inability to close the eye. This puts the cornea at risk from severe dry eye sequelae. Aggressive lubrication is indicated in these patients, who may require their eye to be taped closed at night or a temporary tarsorrhaphy in extreme cases (Feldon, 1989).

SUMMARY

Diagnosis and management of geriatric ocular disease is an important part of the optometric practice. Proper diagnosis is the first stage in helping these patients. Once the diagnosis is made, patients should be informed about their condition and how it can affect them. The doctor and patient should establish goals for therapy centering on the patient's vision, health, and comfort. Then a practical approach to achieving these goals should be developed. Many therapies for ocular disease require the patient's participation, and well-informed patients who are involved in the decisions about their own care are the best participants.

REFERENCES

Alexander LJ. Variations in physician response to consultation requests for Hollenhorst plaques. J Am Optom Assoc. 1992; 63:326–32.

Arffa RC. Grayson's Diseases of the Cornea (3rd ed). St. Louis, C.V. Mosby, 1991.

Bajandas FJ, Kline LB. Neuro-ophthalmology Review Manual (3rd ed). Thorofare, NJ, Slack, 1988.

Branch Vein Occlusion Study Group. Argon laser photocoagulation for macular edema in branch vein occlusion. Am J Ophthalmol 1984; 99:271–282.

Branch Vein Occlusion Study Group. Argon laser photocoagulation for prevention of neovascularization and vitreous hemorrhage in branch vein occlusion. Arch Ophthalmol 196; 104:34–41.

Bressler NM, Bressler SB, Fine SL. Age-related macular degeneration. Surv Ophthalmol 1988; 32:375–413.

Byer NE. Long term natural history of lattice degeneration of the retina. Ophthalmology 1989; 96:1396–1402.

Byer NE. The natural history of asymptomatic retinal breaks. Ophthalmology 1982; 89:1033–1039.

Catania LJ. Primary Care of the Anterior Segment. East Norwalk, CT, Appleton and Lange, 1988.

Diabetic Retinopathy Study Group. Photocoagulation treatment of proliferative diabetic retinopathy. Ophthalmology 1981; 88:583–600.

Early Treatment for Diabetic Retinopathy Group. Early photocoagulation for diabetic retinopathy. Ophthalmology 1991; 98:766–785.

Epstein DL. Chandler and Grant's Glaucoma (3rd ed). Philadelphia, Lea and Febiger, 1986.

Feldon SE. Neuro-ophthalmology. San Francisco, American Academy of Ophthalmology, 1989.

Gass JDM. Macular Diseases (3rd ed). St. Louis, C.V. Mosby, 1987.

Griffith DG, Salasche SJ, Clemons DE. Cutaneous Abnormalities of the Eyelid and Face. New York, McGraw-Hill, 1987.

Katowitz JA. Orbit, Eyelids and Lacrimal System. San Francisco, American Academy of Ophthalmology, 1990.

Kelly, WN. Textbook of Internal Medicine. Philadelphia, J.B. Lippincott, 1989.

McCulley JP. Blepharoconjunctivitis. Int Ophthalmol Clin 1984 24:65–77.

McCulley JP, Dougherty JM, Deneau DG. Classification of chronic blepharitis. Ophthalmology 1983; 89:1173–1180.

Ritch R, Shields MB, Krupin T. The Glaucomas. St. Louis, C.V. Mosby, 1989.

Ryan, SJ. Retina. St. Louis, C.V. Mosby, 1989.

Schepens CL. Retinal Detachment. Philadelphia, W.B. Saunders, 1983.

Shields MB. A Study Guide for Glaucoma. Baltimore, William and Wilkins, 1992.

7

Geriatric Low Vision Rehabilitation

Joseph H. Maino

Approximately one in twenty people in America is visually handicapped; consequently, it is not uncommon for the optometric patient to have some type of permanent visual loss. Fortunately, there have been tremendous improvements in many areas of low vision rehabilitation. Companies such as Eschenbach, Cobern, Telesensory Systems, and Designs for Vision have developed numerous optical, nonoptical, and electronic devices to help restore vision function and minimize the patient's handicap. Government and nongovernment groups such as the Department of Veterans Affairs and the New York Lighthouse for the Blind have developed equipment, evaluation and training procedures, and organizational approaches for the rehabilitation of persons who are visually handicapped. Numerous professional educational opportunities are available through the Association of Schools and Colleges of Optometry, American Academy of Optometry, and New York Lighthouse for the Blind. Finally, more funding resources are becoming available to help pay for the services and devices.

Because of these developments, geriatric low vision rehabilitation services can now be incorporated into the optometric practice. This chapter presents a discussion on adding low vision rehabilitation services to the vision care armenmatarium.

THE NEED

The needs of our elders who have a visual handicap can no longer be ignored. First, there has been and will continue to be an unrelenting increase in the number of older Americans. In 1890 the average life expectancy in the United States was 47; however, by 1986, that life expectancy had increased to 75! This represents a 28-year increase in life expectancy in less than a century. Second, elders now constitute a larger proportion of the population than ever before. In 1900 only 3% of Americans were 65 years old or older. Today more than 12% of our citizens are over 65. In fact, more than 15,000 Americans celebrated their 100th birthday last year!

Recently, Crews looked at the data from the 1984 National Center for Health Statistics (NCHS) Supplement on Aging and projected the growth in the number of severely visually impaired Americans from 1950 through 2030 (Table

7-1). The prevalence rate for severe visual impairment (the inability to read newsprint with best spectacle correction) is 4.7% for those between ages 65 to 75, 9.9% for those between ages 75 to 84, and 25% for those aged 85 and older. His analysis indicates that by the year 2000 there will be more than three million people over the age of 65 with need for low vision rehabilitation services. If the definition of visual impairment is broadened slightly to include "blindness in one or both eyes or any other trouble seeing," by the turn of the century almost five million people will need low vision rehabilitation services (Crews, 1993). These numbers indicate a great social responsibility but also a unique market for optometric low vision rehabilitation services and products.

THE PATIENT

Patients who are older and multiply impaired have more chronic health problems including arthritis, loss of hearing, hypertension, cardiac disease, and orthopedic abnormalities (Kirchner and Phillips, 1988; Kirchner and Peterson, 1988). The combination of aging changes and multiple physical impairments can lead to isolation, depression, and deconditioning (Brummel-Smith, 1990). As a matter of fact, older, severely visually handicapped Americans are much more likely to suffer multiple impairments than those without vision loss. Table 7-2 shows data from the 1984 NCHS Supplement on Aging demonstrating that elders between ages 65 to 74 are three times more likely to have problems with mobility. Arthritis, cardiovascular disease, and hypertension are also significantly increased (Havlik, 1984).

Although many patients who are older and severely visually impaired suffer from multiple age-related diseases and impairments, each individual is unique. A disease or impairment does not automatically lead to a handicap. In 1980 the World Health Organization (WHO) set forth an elegant model describing the relationships between impairment, disability, and handicap. Figure 7-1 describes how disease, disability, and handicap relate to each other.

The optometrist is in a unique position to have a positive impact at all the levels in the WHO model. For example, an older patient may experience vision loss because of dry, age-related macular degeneration (impairment); by diagnosing the problem the optometrist can help prevent additional loss and counsel the patient concerning prognosis and treatment. The patient's reduced vision may result in the inability to read a menu or walk safely, resulting in a disability; consequently, the patient avoids going out to dinner with friends, thus producing a handicap. Low vision rehabilitation can restore the ability to function and reduce the impact of the patient's disability, thereby minimizing the handicap.

THE REHABILITATIVE PROCESS

Low vision rehabilitation of the geriatric patient is different from the low vision care of the younger patient. Older individuals typically present with age-related *and* disease-related reductions in their ability to function. These changes

Table 7-1 The Prevalence of Severely Visually Impaired Americans, 1950–2030

	1950	1960	1970	1980	1990	2000	2010	2020	2030
65–74	395,500	516,900	585,000	732,300	863,500	857,400	988,800	1,455,700	1,691,400
75–84	324,500	458,700	606,300	765,200	983,400	1,189,700	1,528,800	1,662,800	2,032,300
85+	144,300	232,300	353,300	560,000	813,500	1,155,500	1,528,800	1,662,800	2,032,300
Total	863,300	1,207,900	1,544,600	2,057,500	2,660,400	3,202,600	3,726,200	4,548,400	5,850,900

From Crews, JE. The demographic, social, and conceptual contexts of aging and vision loss. JAOA 1993; 64:10; with permission.

Table 7-2 Prevalence of Functional and Medical Impairments in Visually Handicapped Individuals

	65–74 Years Old		85+ Years Old	
	No Visual Impairment	Visual Impairment	No Visual Impairment	Visual Impairment
Difficulty walking	12.3	33.1	39.0	52.9
Difficulty getting outside	4.4	18.4	28.9	46.2
Difficulty getting in and out of a bed or chair	5.8	17.8	19.3	24.4
Arthritis or rheumatism	49.2	66.88	53.3	57.1
Cardiovascular disease	11.3	27.9	25.0	45.0
Hypertension	42.6	55.1	39.7	54.6

From Crews JE: The demographic, social, and conceptual contexts of aging and vision loss. JAOA 1993; 64:10; with permission.

not only affect vision but may also result in impaired cognitive abilities, mobility problems, social problems, and chronic health problems. Consequently, rehabilitation of these patients is a multifaceted, multifactorial process.

To meet a patient's needs the optometrist must diagnose and stabilize the ocular disease, prevent secondary problems, restore lost vision function, help the patient to adapt to his or her environment or recommend changes in the environment, and help the patient's family and friends adapt to the new situation. Low vision rehabilitation services include the low vision prosthetic device evaluation, prescription of devices, training, counseling, orientation and mobility, and rehabilitation teaching. Obviously, optometric low vision care is much more than a refractive service.

The best way to meet the needs of a person with vision loss is through a team approach. A team may be interdisciplinary or multidisciplinary in nature.

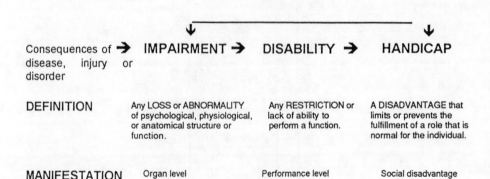

	IMPAIRMENT →	DISABILITY →	HANDICAP
Consequences of → disease, injury or disorder	IMPAIRMENT	DISABILITY	HANDICAP
DEFINITION	Any LOSS or ABNORMALITY of psychological, physiological, or anatomical structure or function.	Any RESTRICTION or lack of ability to perform a function.	A DISADVANTAGE that limits or prevents the fulfillment of a role that is normal for the individual.
MANIFESTATION	Organ level	Performance level	Social disadvantage

Figure 7-1 Models of disablement. *From* WHO.

The multidisciplinary team works in a consulting relationship with reports and telephone consultations to convey information about the patient. The interdisciplinary team, on the other hand, typically works as a group in the same physical setting, meeting there to discuss the patient's rehabilitation plan. Most optometrists start out doing low vision care in a multidisciplinary environment, routinely collaborating with a wide array of health care providers including physicians, rehabilitation teachers, occupational therapists, recreational therapists, physical therapists, orientation and mobility specialists, social workers, and so on. All of these providers also represent an excellent source of referrals for primary care patients to the practice.

THE OFFICE

The optometric office should be scrutinized for accessibility. Can wheelchair and walker patients easily go from the parking lot to the check-in desk? It may be necessary to install ramps, widen doors, and so on to broaden access for those with mobility problems. Are the seats of the chairs in the reception area at an appropriate height and do the chairs have arms so the older patient can get into and out of them easily? Does the reception area have space for wheelchairs? Are the bathrooms accessible to the handicapped? Recent ADA legislation provides architectural guidelines. Contact your local government or rehabilitation agency for additional information.

Look at the office walls, floors, lighting, and furniture. Is there good contrast? Is the floor made of nonskid material? Can wheelchairs roll easily on the carpet? Is the illumination adequate for reading forms? Is large print reading material available in the waiting room? Can wheelchair patients reach the top of the check-in desk? Can the elevator buttons be reached by someone sitting in a wheelchair? Older patients can have hearing problems; is a portable hearing aid* available?

Look at the area that will be used for the low vision examination and rehabilitation. It may be necessary to set aside a separate part of the office for low vision evaluation and training unless one of the examination rooms can be adapted. Is there space in the examination room so a family member or a friend can accompany the patient? Is there enough space to store all the low vision diagnostic and training equipment?

THE STAFF

Regardless of the level of rehabilitation services offered, staff will need additional education to make sure they can meet the needs of the older, visually impaired patient. This may take the form of continuing formal education such as that provided through the American Academy of Optometry, American Opto-

---

*A small, inexpensive, portable hearing aid, **The LISTENAIDER,** can be purchased from Nasta Industries, Inc., 10075 Sandmeyer Lane, Philadelphia, PA 19116

metric Association, American Academy of Ophthalmology, The Lighthouse Inc. in New York City, or the Pennsylvania College of Optometry in Philadelphia. On the job training is also very important.

Staff must come to grips with the idea of working with older, visually handicapped patients. Their own feelings toward aging and blindness must be considered. Their ideas will be valuable when making office modifications to eliminate or minimize obstacles to patient care.

The optometrist may want to add a low vision rehabilitation therapist to the staff. This could be a person with a master's degree in blind rehabilitation or an occupational therapist with additional education in training the visually impaired. The low vision rehabilitation therapist could work in the office part time and/or perform home training in the use of the prescribed optical and nonoptical aids as well as in activities of daily living and basic mobility skills.

THE ROUTINE

To smoothly integrate geriatric low vision services into the practice it is important to take time to look at the office routine. Some practitioners prefer to block out a portion of the work week just for low vision. Many older patients like early morning appointments. If working family members or friends will be providing transportation, consider Saturday low vision appointments.

Consider referral criteria, too. Practitioners new to low vision may prefer to limit patients to those with visual acuity better than 20/200. Many of these individuals are helped with simple low vision aids and a minimal amount of training. Consider who will be referring patients. Local optometrists and ophthalmologists should be informed of new low vision services, along with city, state, and federal organizations for aging and the blind.

Consider the type of information needed from the referring doctors and agencies. It is important to have up-to-date eye and medical data to adequately evaluate patients, and sending the patient a pre-low vision evaluation history form is recommended (Appendix 7-1 and Appendix 7-2). This form will answer many questions concerning the patient's eye and medical history, and can also be used to help the patient formulate specific low vision goals to be worked on during the examination and subsequent training. Several authors have discussed the use of low vision forms and have provided numerous examples to be adapted as needed (Hood and Seidman, 1992; Freeman and Jose, 1991). Use large print whenever possible. Have large-print business cards made up. Patients will notice the extra efforts made on their behalf.

THE EQUIPMENT

To properly perform the low vision refraction, the optometrist needs a good, lightweight trial frame; hand-held Jackson Cross Cylinders (JCC) $(+/-0.50,$

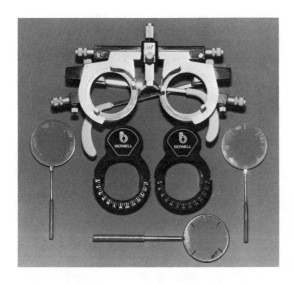

Figure 7-2 Basic equipment needed to perform a low vision refraction includes a trial frame; +/−0.50, +/−1.00, and +/−1.50 JCCs, and Halberg clips.

+/−1.00, and +/−1.50); and corrected curve or full diameter trial lenses. Other useful equipment includes Halberg clips, +/−1.00 confirmation flippers, pinhole, retinoscopy bars and stenopeic slit (Figure 7-2).

Appropriate distance acuity charts include the Feinbloom Distance Number Acuity Chart, Bailey-Lovie Chart, Lighthouse Symbol Cards, and Bailey Hi-Low Contrast Chart (Figure 7-3). These charts are available through Designs for Vision, Lighthouse Low Vision Products, and the Multi-media Center at the University of California, School of Optometry, at Berkeley. These acuity charts require proper illumination. A standard floor goose-neck medical lamp, with a 75 to 100 Watt bulb, can be placed to maximize illumination and minimize glare.

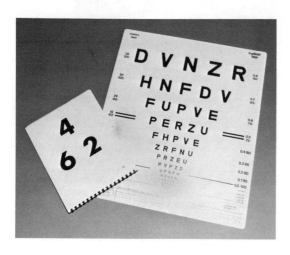

Figure 7-3 Distance acuity charts.

Special near acuity and reading charts are also needed (Figure 7-4). The Lighthouse Near Acuity Chart is used to determine the initial dioptric power required to read standard print (about 20/50). Once that diopter power is known, determine the reading acuity with the Lighthouse Reading Acuity Cards, which use continuous text from 10M to 1M print. These charts also are available from the Lighthouse Low Vision Products department.

The best way to determine the power and type of low vision diagnostic optical and nonoptical aids required is to first determine the kind of patient to be served. Practitioners new to low vision rehabilitation should initially limit patients to those with better than 20/200 visual acuity. Patients at this level typically do well with simple hand and stand magnifiers of +20.00 D or less and hand-held telescopes of less than 4X. (Appendix 7-3 lists basic low vision aids for the optometrist and Appendix 7-4 includes distributors of low vision aids.) As expertise grows, the optical and nonoptical low vision armenmatarium can be expanded.

Low Vision Prosthetic Devices

The four groups of basic low vision optical aids include high plus spectacles, stand magnifiers, hand magnifiers, and telescopes. Spectacles are the most commonly prescribed low vision prosthetic device. Advantages include large reading field and the ability to have both hands free to hold the reading material. A fixed focus and abnormally short working distance are the primary disadvantages.

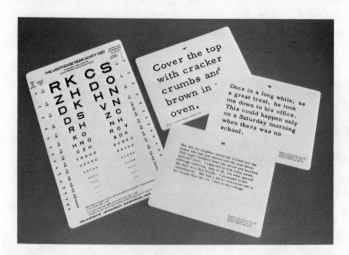

Figure 7-4 The Lighthouse Near Acuity Test *(left)* makes determining the near add needed to read standard print (1M) easy. The Lighthouse Reading Acuity Cards are used to determine the reading acuity *(right)*.

These low vision aids are available in many forms including regular and aspheric lenses, aspheric microscopic lenses, doublets, prism half-eyes, and high plus bifocals and trifocals. A diagnostic spectacle low vision trial set containing prism half-eye, high plus aspheric, and microscopic glasses can be obtained from the Lighthouse Low Vision Product service.

Spectacle low vision aids are best for sustained reading activities. Older patients initially tend to reject the close working distance, but with proper training the patient eventually learns to use and appreciate these low vision aids. The most common mistake made by the low vision clinician when initially presenting this aid is to have the patient move the reading material from a customary working distance *in* toward the nose. A patient will more easily accept high plus spectacles if he or she holds the reading material close to the nose and slowly moves it *away* until the print is in focus.

Hand magnifiers are versatile, simple aids that work well for the patient who cannot adapt to a close working distance (Figure 7-5). The primary benefit of a hand magnifier is an eye to lens working distance that is independent of the lens power. When using the hand magnifier the patient typically uses the distance correction (not the bifocal). The hand magnifier can also be used when a patient is being trained to use a high plus spectacle reading prescription. The patient can be taught to gradually move the hand magnifier and reading material closer to the eye, thus increasing the field of view such that it approaches that of a comparable high plus spectacle lens. Many patients like the increased field of view and eventually request reading glasses.

If a patient has a hand tremor, stand magnifiers may prove beneficial (see Figure 7-4). To reduce aberration these devices have the lens set such that the emerging rays are divergent; consequently, an accommodative effort is required to focus the image. The presbyopic, aphakic, or pseudophakic patient must use a bifocal to focus the light. Keep in mind that the power of the add cannot be

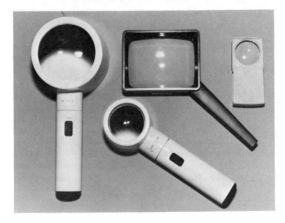

Figure 7-5 Simple hand and stand magnifiers help many elderly patients read the newspaper, thread needles, and so on.

more than that required to focus the stand magnifier's diverging light or the image will be blurred.

Many older patients enjoy using telescopic aids for such activities as spotting and watching television (Figure 7-6). Hand-held telescopes are routinely used to spot bus numbers and street signs. It is not uncommon for the elderly individual who is alone to use the telescope to read the menu that is behind the restaurant counter in fast food restaurants. "Spectacle" telescopes such as the Eschenbach Spectacle Binocular for distance or Walters flip-down telescope are good for watching television or movies. The patient must be cautioned not to walk around while wearing these devices. For patients who need a prescription spectacle-mounted telescopic system consider bioptic telescopes from Designs for Vision, BITA, Ocutek, and Keeler. Hand-held telescopes and spectacle-like telescopes have limited use for patients with hand or head tremors.

Other categories of low vision prosthetic devices include illumination filters, nonoptical aids, electronic low vision aids, and various lamps and illumination controls. For more in-depth information on the characteristics of these as well as other aids mentioned in this chapter, refer to the standard texts listed under "Additional Reading" at the end of this chapter.

It is important to establish a loaner and refund program to give the patient an opportunity to fully evaluate the prosthetic device. Many doctors simply provide a pro-rated reimbursement determined by the length of time the patient has the aid. For example, if the device is returned within 2 weeks, some provide a full refund. On the other hand, if it has been used more than 4 weeks, no refund will

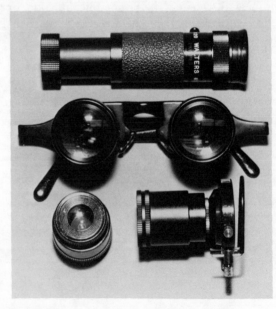

Figure 7-6 Telescopes are useful for spotting and watching television.

be given. Whatever method is used, make sure the patient fully understands the refund policy.

THE EXAMINATION
History and Goals

Geriatric low vision rehabilitation begins even before the patient is seen. A pre-evaluation history and goals questionnaire should be mailed to the patient before the appointment. Freeman and Jose (1991) list suggested questions for the low vision history, and Appendix 7-1 includes a form of questionnaire. In some instances it may be better to have the technician do a prerehabilitation telephone interview (Appendix 7-2). A great deal of time is saved by having the history and goals completed before the evaluation.

These questionnaires give the patient time to think about goals and needs before the appointment. Make sure to encourage patients to bring their own specific reading material or crafts with them so the low vision device for that task can be properly evaluated.

On the day of the low vision evaluation go over the patient's history, paying particular attention to goals. For example, if the patient wants to read, take the time to find out exactly what it is he or she wants to read. One device for reading the newspaper and another one for reading a crossword puzzle may be prescribed.

The Field Evaluation

Tangent screen or Amsler grid testing can help establish guidelines for eccentric fixation training or for orientation and mobility training. The tangent screen provides information about the patient's central thirty degrees, whereas the Amsler grid detects small field defects within the central ten degrees. The optometrist may find the Freeman Functional Near Field Chart valuable when evaluating the patient for scotomata around fixation (Freeman and Jose, 1991).

Patients with central scotomas may have difficulty locating the tangent screen small fixation target. To help the patient fixate, place two strips of white tape over the fixation target such that the strips form an "X." Then simply instruct the patient to look at the point where the two lines would intersect. Another technique is to place a 3 × 5 card in the area of the blind spot and have the patient maintain it as "not seen" while testing.

Keep in mind that any scotoma near fixation will reduce reading speed. If the scotoma is to the right of fixation, reading speed will be reduced because the patient will have difficulty seeing the next word in the sentence. When the scotoma is to the left of fixation the patient may have difficulty finding the next line of print. The former problem may be solved by having the patient hold the reading material at an angle, whereas the latter problem is managed by having the patient use a finger as a guide.

The Distance Low Vision Refraction

The low vision refraction is the foundation on which the entire low vision rehabilitation process is built. Do not assume that the patient's current prescription is adequate. It is not uncommon to find out that those old glasses really belong to Aunt Bessie and not to the patient!

If the patient's old prescription is current, simply clip on Halberg clips and do an over-refraction. If additional cylinder is found, the glasses + over-refraction can be placed in a lensometer and neutralized in normal back-vertex fashion.

Retinoscopy can be tried, but often in the elderly patient the reflex is poor due to cataracts or some other opacity; consequently, the retinoscopy reflex is difficult to neutralize. If media opacities are present try using radical retinoscopy. This retinoscopy technique lets the examiner move as close to the eye as is necessary to obtain a reflex. Once the reflex is neutralized the working distance is measured and its dioptric value subtracted from the retinoscopy finding.

For pseudophakic patients start with keratometry. Place this minus cylinder into the trial frame at the appropriate axis, then add enough plus in the rear well to produce a sphero-equivalent of plano. Also start with keratometry when evaluating aphakic patients but use only two thirds of the cylinder and add a +11.00 to the rear lens well. Remember, these are just rough starting points; it is necessary to refine the refraction.

The distance low vision refraction begins with the starting lenses placed in the trial frame and the trial frame gently placed on the patient's face. Adjust the pupillary distance to place the trial lens optical center in front of the patient's pupil. The distance test chart is typically placed at 10 ft (3 m) and illuminated so the optotypes are seen easily without glare. Examination room illumination is also reduced.

With the left eye occluded make an initial assessment of distance visual acuity for the right eye. This entrance visual acuity is used to determine what pair of plus-minus spherical lenses can be used to refine the prescription. Keep in mind that the worse the acuity, the stronger the lenses must be for the patient to notice a difference. For example, if the patient's visual acuity is 20/50, then +/−0.50 lenses will probably elicit the desired response; however, if visual acuity is 20/400, then +/−2.00 D may be required.

First, place the plus lens in front of the right eye. Ask if the letters are seen better with the lens or without it (Figure 7-7). Be sure to give the patient plenty of time to make a decision. Remember, as one gets older, reaction time slows down. Additionally, if the patient is using eccentric fixation, it may take a while to find the letters. If the letters are improved with the plus lens, then increase the lens power until first blur is noted. If there is no improvement, then test using minus lenses.

Once the spherical power is obtained, then the cylinder axis and power must be determined. When visual acuity is 20/70 or better, use the +/−0.50 JCC to determine the cylinder power and axis. If the acuity is worse than 20/70, use the +/−1.00 or +/−1.50 JCC. In the event the starting lenses do not have an

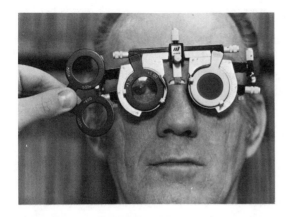

Figure 7-7 When determining the spherical refraction, hold two lenses to help streamline the process. Photograph courtesy of Jeff Ellenwood.

astigmatic correction, a quick method to determine if cylinder is needed is to hold the JCC oriented with the minus axis (red dot) at 180° in front of the eye while asking if the letters are clearer or easier to read. If the letters are better without the lens, rotate the JCC so its minus cylinder is at 90°. If neither of these positions improves the letters, do the same for the 45° and 135° meridians. Obviously, if there is no improvement when the JCC is held in any of the positions, no cylinder is needed. When the cylinder improves vision, add the spherocylinder equivalent to the prescription. For example, if a $+/-1.00$ JCC improved the visual acuity in the JCC minus cylinder axis 90 position, then add $+0.50 -1.00 \times 90$ to the starting lens.

When cylinder is present the first thing to do is determine the axis. Place the handle of the JCC along the starting lens minus lens axis. Flip the JCC, asking if "lens number one or lens number two is better" (Figure 7-8). Rotate the starting lens cylinder in the direction of the red (minus) dot until a reversal is obtained. Once the axis is found rotate the JCC handle such that the red dot is aligned

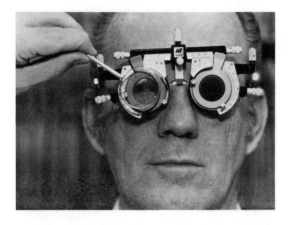

Figure 7-8 To determine the cylinder axis place the handle of the JCC along the axis of the cylinder lens and flip the lens while asking the patient which lens makes the letters easier to read. Rotate the cylinder axis toward the red dot until a reversal is obtained. Photograph courtesy of Jeff Ellenwood.

with the minus axis (Figure 7-9). Again flip the JCC and ask which lens is better. If the patient prefers the red dot, add minus cylinder. If the patient states the black dot improves vision, reduce minus (add plus) power. After the cylinder power and sphere is found, refine the sphere by adding plus or minus lenses to best visual acuity. Once the right eye is done, follow the same procedure for the left eye (Maeda, 1979; Brooks, 1982). During the low vision refraction note any eccentric fixation or the use of a head tilt or turn. This information is useful when training the patient to use the low vision aids and when prescribing spectacle-mounted telescopes.

The Near Low Vision Refraction

The near refraction is the first step to determine the amount of plus required to read standard 1M print (about 20/50). To determine this lens power, occlude the eye with the worse vision and place a +2.50 D lens over the distance prescription. With the Lighthouse Near Acuity Test card held at 40 cm have the patient read down the card until he or she can no longer see the letter. Note the M notation for the last line read. To determine the power required to read 1M print, multiply the M number by 2.5. For example, patients who read down to the 3M line need a +7.50 D add to read 1M single letter text. Test each eye separately as well as binocularly. Occasionally the patient's preferred eye for reading is not the same as the preferred eye for distance. Additionally, some patients must have the eye with the poorer vision occluded to prevent it from interfering with the reading eye.

The reading acuity can be determined by using the Lighthouse Reading Acuity Test Cards, which consist of five reading cards with continuous text printed on both sides. Print size goes from 10M down to 1M. Many patients require more plus to read continuous text than single letter text. In the example just mentioned, the patient probably would require an add of +9.50 D or more to read the acuity cards or newsprint.

Figure 7-9 Cylinder power is found by rotating the JCC handle so the red dot (minus) is along the cylinder lens axis. Again flip the JCC while asking the patient which lens makes the letters clearer. Add minus power if the red dot improves the letters or subtract minus (add plus) if the letters are improved with black dot. Photograph courtesy of Jeff Ellenwood.

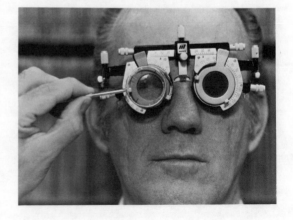

An estimate of the near add also can be obtained by determining the reciprocal of distance or near acuity. For example, if the patient's near acuity is 20/200, at least a +10.00 D must be added for reading 20/50 print (diopters = 1/20/200 = 200/20 = +10.00 D) in the focal plane of the +10.00 D add.

It is important to pay attention to *how* the patient reads when presented with both large and small print. If reading fluency decreases with larger text or magnification, the patient may have a significant field defect. One interesting example of this occurs in patients with central areolar choriodal dystrophy. Many of these patients have a small island of near normal retinal pigment epithelium (RPE) remaining near the fovea that is surrounded by an area of markedly abnormal RPE. The patient literally has a small "island of vision" surrounded by a relative "sea of blindness" (Figure 7-10). The low vision evaluation of these patients is challenging. When magnification or large print is used the image is enlarged over onto the abnormal area of the retina; consequently, this patient typically does worse with magnification than without it!

The Near Low Vision Aid Evaluation

The patient will feel reassured to know that the many trial devices are not necessarily those that will ultimately be prescribed. Reinforce that training to use the devices and an opportunity to work with them on a trial basis will be provided.

Once the dioptric value required for the patient to read continuous text is known, begin to evaluate the patient for a high plus spectacle prescription or a hand or stand magnifier. With high plus spectacles in place, have the patient place the reading material so that it touches the nose and then slowly move it away until the text comes into focus. Start with test material that is at least 1M larger than what might be needed based on the low vision near refraction. Decrease the

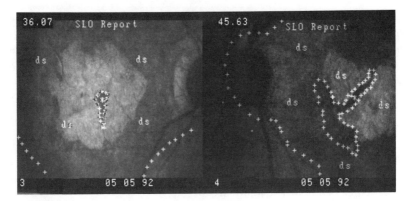

Figure 7-10 The right and left eyes of a patient with central areolar choroidal dystrophy. Note the small island of vision remaining in the right eye. ds = dense scotoma. (Scanning Laser Ophthalmoscope photograph courtesy of Donald Fletcher, MD)

size of the continuous text until the wanted level is reached. If a patient has difficulty reading the desired print size with the initial lens in place, consider increasing the plus and/or adjusting illumination.

When evaluating the patient for a hand magnifier, start with a lens power equal to or slightly greater than that found for the spectacle reading add. Have the patient look through the distance correction while placing the magnifier down on the reading material and then slowly lift the magnifier from the page until the print can be seen. Demonstrate how the hand-magnifier-plus-text can be moved closer to the eye, thus increasing the field of view while leaving the magnification unchanged. If indicated, also evaluate the patient with illuminated systems. Record the near acuity lighting and quality of reading performance; that is, "1.5M with difficulty," "1M and newsprint easily read."

Even if a patient has a good response to hand magnifiers, it is important to take the time to evaluate the response to various stand magnifiers. This is especially true for patients with hand or head tremors. Start with stand magnifiers whose power when added to the patient's bifocal prescription is approximately equal to that required for reading 1M print. Keep in mind that the power of the patient's bifocal cannot be greater than that needed to focus the divergent light coming from the stand magnifier or the text will be blurred. Because of difficulties using external light sources with stand magnifiers, many patients benefit from stand magnifiers with built-in illumination.

The patient can also be evaluated with a host of additional near low vision aids such as telemicroscopes, clip-on loupes, and focusable stand magnifiers. Make sure to take the time to evaluate the patient with actual reading material. Do not assume that they can read their crossword puzzles just because they can read the text on the Lighthouse Reading Acuity Card. Test them actually reading the desired material.

The Distance Low Vision Aid Evaluation

Telescopic low vision devices may be used for movies, television, mobility, sporting events, theater, and sight seeing. Students typically use a telescope for reading the blackboard and watching classroom demonstrations. (Keep in mind that many retired individuals return to school to complete a degree or to learn something new!)

For indoor activities the patient with visually acuity between 20/50 and 20/400 does well with 2X to 4X telescopic systems. If the patient has an outdoor activity such as bird watching, the optometrist may need to use higher power telescopes and binoculars. Telescopic magnification should be titered for the specific task, not simply for a particular acuity. Most patients do not need a telescope to provide 20/20 acuity. For example, to read bus numbers and street signs an acuity of 20/50 is usually acceptable.

Use a 2X or 3X hand-held telescope with a large exit pupil (preferably a Galelean unit) distance evaluation. Prefocus the telescope for the patient. Have the patient look through the distance correction and fixate the distance acuity chart while bringing the telescope up to the eye. Once the chart is located have the patient read a few of the letters and then refocus the telescope to maximize acuity. Evaluate patients with more powerful telescopes as required to meet their goals.

Simple, spectacle-like telescopes such as the 2.5X Selsi Sportglasses and the 3X Eschenbach Spectacle binocular for distance are excellent aids for watching television and movies. If the patient has a moderate or high distance correction, clip-on telescopes from Walters, Selsi, and Eschenbach may be used. Obviously, hand-held and spectacle telescopes are contraindicated for patients with hand or head tremors.

The Illumination Evaluation

Correct lighting is very important for the older patient. The illumination cannot be too bright nor too dim but must be just right for the required task. Glare must also be avoided. Many patients like gooseneck lamps or lamps with adjustable illumination. Patients with age related macular degeneration or diabetic macular edema and near acuity between 20/50 and 20/70 do very well with a moderate (+3.00D to +5.00D) bifocal prescription and a bright light such as Eschenbach's Super-Lite.

Older patients also have more problems with glare and photophobia than younger patients. Fortunately, there is an excellent selection of light filters from which to choose to help them. Fit-over filters such as those from NoIR reduce ultraviolet and infrared transmission, orange filters from Corning heighten contrast, and gray tints are tolerated well by most patients.

The Nonoptical Aid Evaluation

Nonoptical aids may prove more beneficial than optical ones for many visually impaired elders. Do not overlook the use of large print books, newspapers, telephone dials, calculators, clocks, and watches. Large-print playing cards, bingo, and checkers are also available (Figure 7-11).

Some patients do better with talking aids, including talking watches and clocks, calculators, and thermometers. Many older low vision patients also enjoy talking books and audiotapes. Some patients may need high technology products such as computer low vision aids (CLVAs) and closed circuit television (CCTVs). Other "low technology" aids include typoscopes, check writing guides, visors, black felt-tip pens, and wide-lined writing paper. A catalogue containing many of these nonoptical aids can be obtained from the American Foundation for the Blind.

THE TRAINING

Because of the inherent limitations of optical devices (short focal distance, reduced field of view, restricted depth of focus), all patients require at least some instruction in their use. Quillmann (1980) and more recently Freeman and Jose

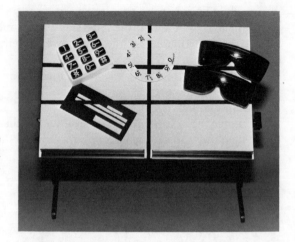

Figure 7-11 Nonoptical low vision prosthetic devices may be even more important than optical aids for some patients. The nonoptical aids above include large print telephone dials, check writing guide, NoIR sunshields, and reading stand.

(1991) have provided guidelines and training exercises to help the patient learn to use the prescribed low vision aids. In the office, delegate much of the training to a properly educated technician. Many metropolitan areas have rehabilitation teachers, orientation and mobility instructors, low vision therapists, or occupational therapists who would be willing to teach the patient in the optometrist's office or in the patient's own home.

In general, for high plus bifocals and microscopes, establishing the proper working distance is most critical. Have the patient hold the reading material close to the nose and slowly back it away until the text is focused. Demonstrate that if the print is held too far away it will be blurred. As the power of the spectacle lens increases, the patient reads better moving the text left to right instead of turning the head.

The patient who will be using a hand-held magnifier must be instructed to look through the distance portion of her glasses. The hand magnifier should be placed on the page and slowly lifted upward until the print is clear and maximally magnified. Demonstrate how the field of view increases as the hand magnifier and print are brought closer to the eye. Remember that trying to read a line of print while keeping everything in focus may take some practice.

Teaching a patient to use a stand magnifier is different from teaching use of a hand magnifier. First of all, a stand magnifier must be used with the patient looking through the bifocal correction. Keep in mind that bifocals above +5.00 do not work, because the image for the stand magnifier is outside the focal distance of the add. Many patients find reading with a stand magnifier easier if they also use a reading stand.

Telescopes are one of the most complicated device to learn how to use. The patient must locate the object of interest, aim the telescope, focus the telescope, and track the target. To complicate the process, as magnification is increased, field of view and image brightness decrease while apparent motion increases. In the author's experience, older patients rarely use telescopes above 6X.

THE FOLLOW-UP EVALUATION

Proper follow up is the key to success in low vision. It may take the form of an office visit, telephone call, or home consultation and can be performed by you or a member of your low vision rehabilitative team. A follow-up program lets you determine if patients require additional training or different low vision aids to accomplish their goals. It also reassures patients that you and your staff want them to succeed.

Follow up is an ongoing process. The time between visits is determined by the stability of the ocular disease, proficiency of the patient in using the aids, characteristics of the aids prescribed, and future needs of the patient.

THE LOW VISION FEE

Rehabilitation of the partially sighted geriatric patient is a complex, time-intensive endeavor. Fortunately, comprehensive low vision care is a legitimate rehabilitative health care service and as such is medicare-reimbursable when "medically necessary and reasonable." To be considered a "medical necessity" functional deficits must exist that low vision rehabilitation can reduce or eliminate, such as safety dependence and/or activities of daily living dependence. These services are deemed "reasonable" if there is a justifiable expectation that therapy will have a significant impact in improving the patient's level of functioning. Keep in mind that medicare will only pay for rehabilitation services provided by a licensed health care practitioner. It will not pay for therapy provided by your optometric technician or a vision rehabilitation therapist. Because physical and occupational therapists are licensed professionals, medicare will pay if the rehabilitation therapy is prescribed and supervised by an optometrist or physician.

Billing for low vision rehabilitation services should list as the primary diagnosis the visual impairment level (Blindness Both Eyes—369.00, Low Vision Both Eyes—369.20, and so on), whereas the secondary diagnosis is the ocular disease (e.g., Retina Degeneration Macular Non-exudative—362.51). Because of the complexity involved, a high level evaluation and management (E&M) code may be

---

☐ Report to Consulting Doctor/Agency

COUNSELING   TIME _____ min. (If counseling > 50% of visits)

☐ DIAGNOSIS	☐ TESTS	☐ VISUAL CONCERNS	☐ INSTRUCTIONS/ADAPTATIONS
☐ PROGNOSIS	☐ RESTRICTIONS	☐ COMPLIANCE	☐ RISKS & BENEFITS OF LV Rx
☐ FOLLOW-UP	☐ REHAB THERAPY	☐HOME THERAPY	☐ FAMILY EDUCATION
☐ OTHER			

Figure 7-12   Counseling checklist.

appropriate. The new CPT 99 series take into account the complex history taking, extensive coordination of care, and extended counseling that is often required in low vision rehabilitation.

When determining the codes to use, select one of five levels of E&M service based on three primary components: the patient evaluation (history, examination, and difficulty of decision); contributory aspects of care (counseling and coordination of care); and time. Time is significant when counseling takes up more than 50% of the visit. Documentation is very important. Figure 7-12 shows a checklist that can be used on the examination form to help document the counseling services provided and time spent counseling the patients.

For additional information on billing for low vision rehabilitation services see Fletcher and Weinstock, 1992; Piqueras, 1991; and Fletcher and Weinstock, 1991. Be sure to check with the area medicare intermediary for additional information.

SUMMARY

Every visually impaired geriatric patient represents a unique challenge for the low vision clinician. What works for one patient may not work for another. Fortunately, the optometrist is uniquely trained to manage these patients' ophthalmic, visual, and optical needs. Low vision rehabilitation can help them lead more satisfying and fulfilling lives.

Acknowledgement

I would like to acknowledge Dr. Derrel Taylor for his comments regarding this chapter.

REFERENCES

Brummel-Smith K. Introduction. *In* Kemp B, Brummel-Smith K, Ramsdell JW (eds) Geriatric Rehabilitation. Boston, Little Brown, 1990.

Crews JE. The demographic, social, and conceptual contexts of aging and vision loss. J Am Optom Assoc 1993;64:10.

Fletcher DC, Weinstock FJ. E&M codes for low vision rehabilitation. Argus 1992; August, p 24.

Fletcher DC, Weinstock FJ. How to use CPT codes for low vision rehabilitation. Argus 1991; January, p 16.

Freeman PB, Jose RT. The Art and Practice of Low Vision. Boston, Butterworth-Heinemann, 1991.

Havilik RJ: Aging in the eighties. Impaired senses for sound and light in persons age 65 and over: Preliminary data form the *Supplement on Aging to the National Health Interview Survey: United States*. January–June, 1984. Advance Data, No. 125, September 18, 1986.

Hood CM, Seidman KR. Setting up a low vision practice. *In* Cole RG, Rosenthal BP (eds): Problems in Optometry. Patient and Practice Management in Low Vision 1992,(4)1:107–116.

Kirchner C, Peterson R. Data on visual disability from NCHS, 1977. *In* C Kirchner (ed): Data on Blindness and Visual Impairment in the U.S. (2nd ed). New York, American Foundation for the Blind, 1988, pp 19–24.

Kirchner C, Phillips B. Report of a survey of U.S. low vision services. *In* C Kirchner (ed): Data on blindness and visual impairment in the U.S. (2nd ed). New York, American Foundation for the Blind, 1988, pp 285–293.

Nelson KA. Statistical brief #35: Visual impairment among elderly Americans: Statistics in transition. J Visual Impairment & Blindness 1987; 81:331–334.

Piqueras L. Third party reimbursement of vision rehabilitation services: A historical overview. J Visual Impairment & Blindness 1992; 86(1):10–13.

Quillman RD. Low Vision Training Manual. Kalamazoo, Western Michigan University, 1980.

ADDITIONAL READING

Brooks CW. A systematic method of subjective trial frame refraction. Optom Monthly 1982;8:433–438.

Faye EE. **Clinical Low Vision** (2nd ed). Boston, Little, Brown, 1984.

Fonda G. Management of low vision in the geriatric patient. *In* Kwitko ML, Weinstock FJ (eds): **Geriatric Ophthalmology.** Orlando, Grune and Stratton, 1984, pp 351–379.

Jose, RT. *Understanding Low Vision.* New York, American Foundation for the Blind, 1983.

Lovie-Kitchin JE, Bowman KJ. **Senile Macular Degeneration: Management and Rehabilitation.** Boston, Butterworth-Heinemann, 1985.

Maeda AY. Trial frame refraction. Optom Monthly 1979; 10:122–127.

Mehr EB, Fried AN. **Low Vision Care.** Chicago, Professional Press, 1975.

Rosenbloom AA. Care of the visually impaired elderly patient. *In* Rosenbloom AA, Morgan MW (eds): **Vision and Aging: General and Clinical perspectives.** New York, Professional Press Books, 1986, pp 337–348.

Sloane LL: **Reading Aids for the Partially Sighted: A Systematic Classification and Procedure for Prescribing.** Baltimore, Williams & Wilkins, 1977.

Low Vision Patient Questionnaire

NAME: _____ SEX: M F AGE: _____
BIRTHDATE: _____ PHONE: _____
ADDRESS: _____

General health: Excellent Good Fair; Explain: _____
_____

Mobility: (Circle answer, then comment)
Does patient have a guide dog, cane, or use sighted guide?
Bumps into things? _____ Falls over things? _____
_____

Lighting problems: Does the patient see better in bright light or dim light? Does glare bother the patient? Is the patient sensitive to light? _____
_____

Reading problems (explain): _____
_____

Educational level (years): Grade School _____ High School _____ College _____
Other: _____

Occupation before onset of eye problem: _____
Occupation after onset of eye problem: _____
Current occupation: _____

Interests and/or hobbies: _____
_____

What caused the patient's eye problems? _____
_____

When did the eye problem begin? _____

Can the patient:
Read headlines	Y	N	Sometimes
Read newspaper	Y	N	Sometimes
See photographs	Y	N	Sometimes
Recognize faces	Y	N	Sometimes
Recognize colors	Y	N	Sometimes

Can the patient:

Dial telephone	Y	N	Sometimes
Read price tags	Y	N	Sometimes
Read labels	Y	N	Sometimes
See TV	Y	N	Sometimes
See watch	Y	N	Sometimes

Does the patient currently use magnifiers or other low-vision aids?
Y   N   Sometimes

_____

_____

Does patient have a hearing problem?   Y   N   Sometimes
Comment: _____

Does the patient drive?   Y   N   Sometimes
Comment: _____

Goals:
1 _____
2 _____
3 _____

Who filled out this form: Patient/Relative/Friend/Other

Signature: _____ Date _____

Telephone Low Vision History

Name: _____

SSN: _____

Address: _____

_____

D.O.B.: ___/___/___

Marital Status: M/W/D/S

Consulting Doctor/Agency _____

HISTORY

Eye DX: _____

_____

_____

Med Hx: _____

_____

_____

Meds: _____

_____

_____

Mobility: _____

_____

_____

ADL: _____

_____

Reading: _____

_____

Illum: _____

_____

Other: _____

_____

_____

GOALS

1. _____
2. _____
3. _____
4. _____
5. _____

VISUAL FUNCTION

Can You?	Yes	No	Comments
READ HEADLINES			
READ NEWSPRINT			
SEE PHOTOGRAPHS			
SEE FACES			
SEE COLORS			
DIAL PHONE			
READ PRICE TAGS			
READ LABELS			
READ MED BOTTLES			
SEE TV/MOVIES			
SEE ACROSS STREET			
SEE WATCH			
WRITE CHECK			
SEE FOOD ON PLATE			
OTHER COMMENTS			

LOW VISION AIDS

Do you have/use any of the following?

Magnifiers   Glasses

Large-print Books   Talking Books

Binoculars   Contact Lenses

Tape Recorder   Other

ASSESSMENT   Priority: Yes   No

Motivation: _____   Comments: _____
            _____   _____
            _____   _____
Goals: _____
            _____
            _____

Basic Low Vision Prosthetic Devices

Near Spectacles
  Prism half-eyes +4.00 Diopters to
    +12.00 Diopters
  High Plus Aspheric Lenticular +4.00
    Diopters to +20.00 Diopters
  Microscopic Spectacles 4X to 12X

Hand Magnifiers (HM)
  +3 D Eschenbach Bar Magnifiers
    (with and without red line)
  +3 D Easi View Hands Free
    Magnifier (hangs around neck)
  +5 D B&L Rectangular Illuminated
    and Non-Illuminated HM
  +8 D Coil HM
  +12 D & +20D B&L Packette HM
  +12 D Magna-lite HM
  +12 D Eschenbach Illuminated HM
  +20 D Coil Cataract HM
  +24 D Eschenback Illuminated HM
  +36 D Eschenbach Illuminated HM

Stand Magnifiers (SM)
  +8 D Eschenbach Illuminated SM
  +12 D Eschenbach SM
  +16 D Eschenbach SM
  +12 D Eschenbach Illuminated SM
  +15.6 D Coil Raylight Illuminated
    SM
  +20 D Eschenbach Illuminated SM
  +20 D Coil Large Cataract SM
  +24 D Eschenbach Illuminated SM
  +28 D Coil SM
  +24 D Eschenbach Illuminated SM
  +36 D Eschenbach Illuminated SM

Telescopes
  2.5X Selsi Sportglasses
  3X Eschenbach Spectacle Binoculars
  2.5X Selsi Monocular Telescope
  3X Eschenbach Monocular
    Telescope
  4X Walters Monoclar Telescope
  4X Eschenbach Monocular
    Telescope
  6X Walters Monocular Telescope.
  8X Walters Monocular Telescope

Nonoptical Aids
  Typoscope
  Check writing guide
  Reading stand
  Large-print telephone dials
  Various lamps
  Large-print Readers Digest (sample)
  Large-print book (sample)
  Visorette
  Felt tip pens

Light Filters (LF)
  #101 & #102 NoIR LF
  U40 & U22 NoIR UV Shields
  Various clip-on filters from NoIR &
    Corning (CPF-S & CPF-Dn)

Low Vision Equipment Sources

American Foundation For the Blind
15 West 16th Street
New York, NY 10011
(800) AFBLIND
(212) 620-2000

Bernell Corporation
750 Lincolnway East
Box 4637
South Bend, IN 46634
(800) 348-2225

Coburn Optical Industries, Inc.
P.O. Box 627
1701 South Cherokee Rd
Muskogee, OK 74402
(800) 262-8761

Corning Medical Optics
Corning, NY 14831
(800) 742-5273

Designs for Vision
760 Koehler Ave
Ronkonkoma, NY 11779
(800) 345-4009

Eschenbach Otik of America
25 November Trail
Weston, CT 06883
(203) 227-9409

Keeler Optical
456 Parkway
Broomall, PA 19008
(800) 523-5620
(215) 353-4350

Mattingly International
938 K-A Andreason Dr.
Escondido, CA 92029
(800) 826-4200

NoIR
P.O. Box 159
South Lyon, MI 48178
(800) 521-9746

Lighthouse Low Vision Products
111 East 59th St.
New York, NY 10022
(212) 355-2200

Telesensory Systems
P.O. Box 7455
Mountain View, CA 94039
(800) 227-8418
(415) 960-0960

Walters, Inc.
Suite 126
30423 Canwood St
Agoura Hills, CA 91301
(818) 706-2202

Optelec
4 Lyberty Way
Westford, MA 01886
(508) 392-0707

8

Contact Lenses for the Older Adult

Timothy T. McMahon
Joseph H. Maino

Contact lenses are a commonly overlooked modality for vision correction in older adults, and this oversight often may not be in the best interest of this segment of the population. There are a number of circumstances for which contact lenses are not only suitable for vision correction but are the best method of treating a vision problem. The purpose of this chapter is to provide a sound rationale for contact lenses and to describe the methods for determining the best treatment option in the eye care management of the older adult.

INDICATIONS

Evaluating prospective contact lens wearers begins with an understanding of the indications for their use. These include refractive error, cosmetic concerns, occupational demands, postoperative care, and the need for therapeutic lenses.

Refractive Error

Correction of refractive error is the most common reason for using contact lenses and provides the strongest rationale for prescribing contact lenses for the older adult. The types of refractive errors are similar to those found in a younger population; however, experience has shown that the breakdown percentages of refractive corrections is different in this population (US Department of Health, Education, and Welfare, 1971–72). The relevant refractive categories include anisometropia, myopia, astigmatism, hyperopia, and aniseikonia.

Anisometropia

High amounts of anisometropia are more frequently found in older adults than in young adults or children. This is due primarily to optical density changes of the human crystalline lens and to ocular surgical intervention. The existence of higher dioptric amounts of anisometropia is compounded by the rapid or immediate onset of this refractive error. In these cases correction with contact lenses is often the best treatment option. For interocular differences in refractive error of 3 D or more, contact lenses should be high on the list of treatment options.

Aniseikonia

Aniseikonia is not a common problem in older adults except as it relates to anisometropia. The management of this condition for those without new or progressive changes in refractive error is the same as for young adults. Aniseikonia resulting from changes in refractive error commonly can be eliminated or greatly minimized with the use of contact lenses.

Astigmatism

Astigmatism is a common refractive feature in older adults. This population is relatively unique due to the high frequency of against-the-rule refractions. Commonly this is found with a small amount of with-the-rule corneal astigmatism and, to a lesser extent, in spherical corneas. The increase in the frequency in against-the-rule astigmatism found in older adults is attributed principally to greater lenticular astigmatism.

Myopia

Myopia is very common in the elderly. In fact, its frequency is similar to, or slightly higher, than that for younger adults. "Once a myope, always a myope—unless iatrogenically or pathologically altered" is a good rule of thumb to follow. The reasons for correcting myopia with a contact lens are the same as those for younger adults: visual acuity, occupational or avocational demands, cosmetic concerns, or spectacle intolerance.

Hyperopia

Hyperopia is very common. The frequency of hyperopic prescriptions increases with age (US Department of Health, Education, and Welfare, 1971–72). The increase in frequency is often misinterpreted as representing a shift in the population toward a greater prevalence of hyperopia. Actually, the population is not becoming more hyperopic; rather, the hyperopic portion of the population, which has always represented the majority, increasingly requires optical correction with increasing age. A decrease in the amplitude of accommodation incumbent with aging yields a higher demand for visual correction as the latent component of hyperopia becomes manifest. This higher demand for visual correction translates to a higher portion of the total population who potentially would benefit from contact lenses.

Cosmetic Concerns

Older adults have significant cosmetic concerns, although their motivation may be different than those of younger age groups. In a recent study comparing the satisfaction with eyeglasses, dentures, and hearing aids among the elderly, glasses finished in the middle behind dentures (Smedley et al., 1989). In the 391 patient sample, of which 137 were spectacle users, 14% were dissatisfied with their glasses, and 34% who were somewhat satisfied made negative comments concerning their spectacle use. Equally informative was the fact that only 14%

were very satisfied with their spectacles. Although it is the authors' clinical experience that concern about appearance as a motivator for contact lens wear decreases with increasing age, the clinician should not assume that for all older persons desiring "good looks" is insufficient reason for lens wear.

Occupational or Avocational Demands

Occupational or avocational reasons for wearing contact lenses are not common, in our experience, for the older adult. When this becomes an issue, it usually involves a patient with a low ametropic refractive error who continues to have difficulties using reading glasses.

Postsurgical Optical Correction

The frequency of need for contact lens correction after surgery has decreased over the past decade with the advent of the intraocular lens. Although aphakia is rapidly diminishing as an ophthalmic condition, a number of aphakic patients will continue to need suitable aphakic contact lenses as well as clinicians with the necessary expertise to fit them. Other ocular surgical procedures that represent indications for contact lens fitting include penetrating keratoplasty, epikeratoplasty, and refractive surgery with residual error; retinal detachment repair with resultant anisometropia; and surgically altered pupils.

Bandage and Therapeutic Lenses

Bandage lenses and other types of therapeutic lenses are not commonly needed by the older population when compared with the whole population, but they are more often needed for the elderly than for younger age groups.

PRECAUTIONS

Some conditions require precaution in the fitting of contact lenses. They are listed in Table 8-1, and some of them are discussed here, along with other preexisting conditions that can affect contact lens wear.

Dry Eyes

Tear insufficiency is quite common and poses a significant problem for many in the older population (Hamano et al., 1990). Schirmer tear strip measurements or other similar commercially available test measurements should be used routinely to test whether tear production is sufficient to allow contact lens wear. Whether tear film break up time (TBUT) should be measured is questionable. Many authors feel that this measurement is quite important (Andres et al., 1987; Stewart, 1971; MacKeen, 1986). We believe that a qualitative observation of the oily layer of the tear film offers the same information as a timed measurement of a break up

Table 8-1 Precautions in Fitting Contact Lenses.

Symblepharon
Pterygium
Exposure keratitis
Filtering blebs
Diabetes mellitus
Corneal vascularization
Dry eyes
Vernal conjunctivitis
Ocular pemphigoid
Corneal dystrophies
Blepharitis
Poor compliance
Anterior segment inflammatory disease
Bullous keratopathy
Fifth nerve palsy
Corneal scarring

in wetting and integrity of the mucinous layer. In general, fitting of contact lenses in individuals with poor baseline tear film function should be approached cautiously, and the patient should have his or her expectations appropriately downgraded commensurate with the degree of tear insufficiency.

Blepharitis and Meibomian Gland Dysfunction

Anterior blepharitis and meibomian gland dysfunction (MGD) are all too common. These related conditions are a major nuisance for contact lens users, particularly when they are found in combination with dry eyes. The clinician should aggressively treat these conditions in the older patient with contact lenses.

Severe Arthritis

Osteoarthritis is well recognized as a common condition in older persons. This form of arthritis represents a problem when it is severe or when acute inflammation exists. Arthritic hands and neck can make it difficult for the patient to clean, insert, and remove lenses. Rheumatoid arthritis requires a more careful evaluation for lens handling reasons and for intraocular and corneal problems. Uveitis, dry eyes, and corneal vascularization are within the spectrum of problems for this destructive disease. The patient with rheumatoid disease should have more frequent follow-up examinations, including a careful evaluation of tearing levels and conscientious investigation of lens-handling difficulties.

Poor Vision

Poor central vision can be a problem for prospective contact lens patients, primarily due to troubles with handling lenses and the possibility of lens loss. These problems are more frustrating than they are dangerous; however, the clinician should also be concerned about whether patients with low vision have limited travel capabilities that could prevent them from reaching suitable optometric or medical attention in the event of a contact lens-related ocular emergency. This concern needs to be weighed by both the patient and the practitioner.

Mental Status and Memory

In elderly persons, short-term memory status and cognitive condition must be considered. Organic brain syndrome and Alzheimer's disease are not uncommon among those aged 70 years or older. The concern regarding contact lenses is obvious. Contact lens wear requires either the patient or an extremely attentive significant other or caretaker to manage the cleaning and care of lenses, insertion and removal, appropriate wearing schedules, timely follow-up visits to the doctor, and appropriate behavior in the event of an emergency or complication. There should be a substantial need for contact lenses before they are seriously considered as a vision correction option in anyone whose mental status may be compromised.

Monocularity

Monocularity requires caution on the part of the clinician. Even when a patient has both eyes, contact lenses carry a greater risk than wearing glasses. Not only must the medical risks associated with contact lens wear be considered, but also the loss of protection provided by spectacle lenses. Therefore, when a practitioner is considering contact lenses for patients who have lost vision in one eye, a careful appraisal of the risk to benefit ratio for contact lens wear is necessary.

Strabismus

Strabismus merits special mention rather than a precautionary status. Three issues are important in strabismic cases relative to contact lens wear. The first is cosmetic appearance. Pay direct attention to the appearance of the patient with and without glasses. If the strabismus is more apparent without glasses, trial fit with a contact lens having power very close to what the patient needs and then reevaluate the ocular alignment. If the appearance is improved without spectacles, do the same thing, but expect a better cosmetic outcome. The second issue is diplopia. Even well-imbedded "suppressors" can become diplopic with significant alterations to the alignment of their suppression area. Actively inquire about diplopia as the examination, testing, and lens fitting proceeds. The third issue relates to the relative monocular status of some strabismic patients. Strabismic individuals who are functionally monocular need to be considered monocular and appropriately evaluated.

CONTRAINDICATIONS

Certain ophthalmic conditions provide sufficient reason to recommend against fitting new contact lenses as well as to discontinuing use of current contact lenses (Table 8-2); (Dart, 1988; Omerod, 1989). There are circumstances, however, such as the use of bandage lenses, where contact lens use may be indicated in the presence of these ocular diseases. The conditions can be divided into five general categories: corneal surface disease, including inflammatory disease; infections of the cornea or conjunctiva; keratitis sicca; severe blepharitis; and patient noncompliance.

Corneal Surface Disease

Corneal surface disease represents those problems in which involvement of the corneal epithelium is evident. This includes recurrent erosions, abrasions, chemical keratitis, basement membrane diseases with epithelial defects, and inflammatory corneal disease. In general, if the epithelium is sick or there is an inflammatory process active in the cornea, avoid prescribing contact lenses unless the lens is being used therapeutically to treat the problem.

Infectious Keratitis or Conjunctivitis

Active infectious diseases of the cornea or conjunctiva are contraindications to contact lens use. Once the infection has resolved, a return to lens wear needs to be determined on a case-by-case basis, taking into consideration need, extent of damage from the infection, risk of future infections, and so on.

Keratitis Sicca

True keratitis sicca, or the pathologically dry eye, is a contraindication to contact lens wear. With this condition, even therapeutic bandage lenses are generally not recommended. If the eye is not wet enough to support its own physical requirements, it will not support a contact lens.

Table 8-2 Contraindications for Fitting Contact Lenses

Inflammatory keratitis
Active infections of the eye or adnexa
Keratoconjunctivitis sicca
Stevens-Johnson syndrome
Corneal vascularization (within 2 mm of visual axis)
Noncompliance

Severe Blepharitis or Meibomian Gland Dysfunction

In severe cases of eyelid disease, whether infectious or not, contact lenses should be avoided. If there is any question of the severity of the condition and the suitability for contact lens wear, it is wise to presume the worst and defer or discontinue lens use until the lid disease is treated.

Patient Noncompliance

Poor compliance is very common among contact lens wearers but infrequently involves actions that may be imminently hazardous to the patient. On the other hand, noncompliance—the absence of compliance—is less common but includes actions or a history of actions that clearly carry significant risk of harm to the patient. This differentiation is not traditional. Most clinicians tend to lump the two classes of bad compliance under the same category. In the authors' opinion poor compliers warrant reinforced instructions, guidance, and closer follow-up examinations, whereas noncompliers should not be fit with lenses or should stop wearing them. In short, if a patient cannot or will not act responsibly, the clinician should not fit that person with lenses and should discourage future use of contact lenses until noncompliant behavior can be eliminated.

HISTORY

A detailed case history is necessary for a successful outcome in fitting contact lenses. Information should be obtained from a prospective contact lens wearer pertaining to (1) motivation and compliance, (2) ocular and systemic medical history, (3) optical history, and (4) occupational and environmental history.

Motivation and Compliance

Motivation is a difficult entity to ascertain accurately. In general, a moderate to high degree of motivation is desired because of day-to-day procedures the patient will need to perform and the initial adaptive symptoms that may be experienced. Poor motivation commonly results in patients discontinuing lens wear over time.

Compliance with the instructions given is important for successful lens wear and the lessening of risks associated with lens use. Studies have demonstrated that many patients are poorly compliant. Therefore, a patient with a history of marginal compliance should be discouraged from contact lens wear when other options for visual correction exist.

Ocular and Systemic Medical History

The most important part of the history-taking pertains to the past and present health status of the eye and surrounding structures, as well as the remaining organs and systems. It is useful to divide ocular conditions into two categories:

those in which the clinician can proceed with fitting contact lenses with caution and those in which fitting is considered to be contraindicated, as previously described.

The systemic medical history should concentrate on allergies, medications being taken, diabetes, neurologic or musculoskeletal abnormalities affecting the limbs, and mucous membrane diseases.

Allergy

Allergies to contact lens care products and preservatives are common. This is particularly true for thimerosal, a preservative that has been implicated in a potentially sight-threatening complication, superior limbic keratoconjunctivitis associated with soft lens wear (SLK-SCL). An atopic history is also significant because of the higher failure rate due to lens wear intolerance in these patients.

Medication

Systemic and ocular medications being taken are of potential importance in that some discolor lenses, some alter immunologic activities, some have anesthetic properties, some are toxic to epithelial cells, and others may have mucous membrane drying or lacrimal inhibitory activity. The more common agents of concern are the atropine family of drugs, antihistamines, vasoconstrictors, epinephrine, and topical beta blockers.

Neurologic and Musculoskeletal Disorders

Neurologic and musculoskeletal disorders may be of significance to the contact lens practitioner if the tonicity of the lid musculature or blink responses are affected, corneal hyposensitivity exists, or dexterity of arms or fingers is restricted.

Mucous Membrane Diseases

Disorders of the mucous membranes of the body usually have significant ocular consequences such as keratitis sicca, cul-de-sac foreshortening, symblepharon, and cicatricial entropion. The role of contact lenses is mainly therapeutic in these cases. Cosmetic contact lens use should be discouraged. The role of contact lens wear in cases of mild tear film insufficiency should be determined on a case-by-case basis with some caution.

Optical Needs and History

The visual needs and problems of the patient should be part of any ocular history. Particular attention should be paid to the patient's past experience with optical corrections and any related visual complaints. In many cases, past problems with glasses lead the patient to try contact lens wear. Reviewing this portion of the history may establish whether the patient's expectations are reasonable and optically obtainable.

Most cosmetic contact lens candidates will fit into the following categories, relative to their optical needs and history: (1) the acute (oversensitive) observer, (2) the patient who does not like spectacle frames, (3) the patient with thick spectacle lenses, (4) the athlete, (5) the patient who never has tolerated the visual distortions seen through glasses, (6) the patient with ten pairs of glasses, and (7) the presbyope.

The Acute (Oversensitive) Observer
A person with distinct affective characteristics warrants caution with regard to contact lens fitting. The acute observer tends to direct incredible attention and emotional energy to small changes in refractive errors and vision and may have difficulty adjusting to new glasses or contact lenses. This type of patient can be a good contact lens candidate if expectations for visual acuity are attenuated such that minor fluctuations and obscurations in vision will be expected and accepted.

The Patient Who Does Not Like Spectacle Frames
The most common reason expressed for desiring contact lenses is a dislike for the cosmetics or discomfort of spectacle frames. In general, patients with this motivation can successfully wear contact lenses.

The Patient with Thick Spectacle Lenses
Individuals with moderate to high myopia or high hyperopia generally will prefer the cosmetic and optical improvement of contact lenses to that of glasses. These patients tend to have a strong motivation to succeed in contact lens wear.

The Athlete
The sports enthusiast who wishes or needs to avoid glasses during sports can be a troublesome patient. If contact lenses are to be worn only during sports, the options are limited to hydrogels, due to their greater stability and more flexible wearing schedule. Rigid lenses can be worn for most sports (except swimming) if fit properly. The loss rate may be higher, however, than for hydrogels. Attention should be placed on the magnification change experienced when changing from spectacles to contact lenses. This is very important for those who participate in ball sports, such as tennis, golf, and baseball.

The Patient Who Never Has Tolerated the Visual Distortions Seen Through Glasses
Commonly, patients who demonstrate uncorrected visual acuities between 20/40 and 20/200 do not wear their glasses because they prefer blurred vision to the visual distortions produced by their spectacle lenses. Surprisingly often, these patients have high levels of astigmatism (>2.00 D), a spherical equivalent refraction within 1 D of plano, and at times, meridional amblyopia. Some of these patients do well with contact lenses, but before lenses are ordered, the patient should clearly appreciate an improvement in vision with them. This should be documented by finding at least two lines of improvement above their uncorrected acuity on the visual acuity chart.

The Patient with Ten Pairs of Glasses

Some patients represent one or more of the other categories but are unique in that they maintain a host of spectacles at the ready. Usually the prescriptions are very similar. This group of patients warrants careful attention as to their reason for desiring contact lenses. Often there is a near and/or intermediate distance vision component to their troubles that may not be adequately dealt with by contact lenses.

The Presbyope

Presbyopes who want contact lenses usually do so to avoid using bifocal spectacles or because they are curious about contact lenses or because of occupational/social needs. The first reason is the most common. At present, the options for presbyopic contact lens management are not equal to spectacles in constant, stable, consistent vision, and caution should therefore be used in fitting the presbyope with contact lenses. An accurate assessment of motivation and expectations is necessary to achieve success with this very sizable population of patients.

Occupational and Environmental History

A patient's occupation and environment are interwoven. The importance of these factors to contact lens wear relates to the effect of the occupational activities on blinking rate and the presence of noxious agents coming into contact with the lens and the eye.

Individuals who spend a substantial amount of time reading or looking at a computer screen generally have a prolonged interblink period when the lens surface or lens matrix dries. This leads to foggy vision, discomfort, decreased lens tolerance, and similar symptoms. Attention to tear film volume, quality, and blinking habits is important in predicting suitability for contact lens wear.

Noxious products in one's environment can be adsorbed to or absorbed by the lens. Oils, fumes, and particulate debris all can cause trouble. Soft lenses are exceptionally prone to absorbing oils and fumes. Rigid lenses will absorb some of these, but patients are more likely to complain about particulate debris pumped under the lens via the tear pump.

PHYSICAL EXAMINATION

The initial physical examination of the anterior segment of the eye and its adnexa should include the following:

1. Visual acuity, uncorrected, at distance and near (sV) (snV)
2. Visual acuity, with spectacles, at distance and near (cV) (cnV)
3. Prescription of current glasses (W)
4. Keratometry (K)
5. Manifest refraction and visual acuities with near add if appropriate (M)
6. Tonometry (where appropriate) (Tp or Ta)

7. Slit-lamp examination
8. Schirmer tear testing at 1 minute with application of anesthetic (S)
9. Break up time (BUT) (optional)

The uncorrected vision for a patient is relevant in two respects. First, this measurement serves as an unaltered baseline for potential future comparison and, second, it may serve as a useful indicator of the underlying motivational factors bringing the patient to you for contact lenses. Persons with 3 D of myopia at the initial examination for contact lenses who are not wearing glasses are indicating they cannot or will not use glasses some or all of the time, and equally important, that blur is largely tolerated. The latter information allows for a potentially broader range of lens options to use.

During the slit-lamp examination particular attention should be paid to the quality of the tear film, the lid position and lid margins, conjunctival surface, tarsal conjunctival appearance, blinking pattern (partial or complete), cornea and pupil size.

CHOOSING THE RIGHT MATERIAL

The myriad of available lens materials offers numerous choices to the contact lens practitioner. The lens material should be selected based on individual patient needs and ocular requirements. The practitioner should keep in mind that an 80-year-old contact lens patient has different needs and physical requirements than a 20-year-old patient.

Most older contact lens patients have some form of dry eye, chronic meibomianitis, and/or chronic blepharitis; consequently, the selected contact lens material must be compatible with an abnormal tear composition. Choosing between hydrogel and rigid gas permeable (RGP) lenses is not a straightforward issue. Hydrogel lenses generally are perceived as being more comfortable than RGP lenses but suffer from spoilage and damage problems and probably a true higher incidence of microbial infection in older patients (Tripathi et al., 1980; Tripathi and Tripathi, 1981; Liotet et al., 1983). Rigid lenses, particularly the fluoropolymer designs, offer great optics, deposit resistance, and toughness. Due to its superior optical surface wettability, a fluorosilicone/acrylate material with a low Dk (30–45) is recommended if a rigid material is likely to be tolerated. Aphakes and high hyperopes typically require higher oxygen permeability to deliver sufficient oxygen through a thicker lens. These patients tend to do well with higher Dk fluoropolymer and fluorosilicone/acrylate lenses (Bennett, 1991). In general, our experience has been that many older people with tear insufficiency poorly tolerate any rigid lens and prefer hydrogels despite their shortcomings.

Lid anatomy should also be considered when choosing a lens material. Eyelids become lax with age and have a tendency to pull away from the bulbar surface. Ectropion is also a common problem. Heavy, thick lenses will have a tendency to be displaced inferiorly. Better centration may be obtained in these patients with RGP and hydrogel lenses.

MANAGING PRESBYOPIA

Ever since Benjamin Franklin first invented bifocal spectacles, men and women have been trying numerous methods to avoid wearing them! Current alternatives to bifocal spectacles include bifocal contact lenses, monovision contact lenses, and a combination of contact lenses and reading glasses.

Bifocal Contact Lenses

Practitioners have been prescribing bifocal contact lenses since 1936 (Caplan and Molinari, 1984). The first bifocal contacts were constructed from PMMA. Fortunately, today we have lighter, gas-permeable materials that are better suited for the physiologic demands of the older eye.

Many ocular changes associated with aging influence the selection of the lens material and design. As we age, changes in the lacrimal and meibomian glands, goblet cells, crypts of Henle, and the glands of Zeis, Moll, Wolfring, Krause, and Manz contribute to an altered tear layer. All these changes can lead to chronic dry eyes and an unsuccessful or marginally successful lens fit.

Miosis related to aging also limits the practitioner's choices for lens design. A small, sluggish pupil produces a problem when aspheric or annular bifocal lenses are used. Success with these lenses dictates that the pupillary area needs to be large enough to cover both the distance and near portions of the contact lens. For very small pupils, the practitioner should select a translating, alternating image bifocal design.

Diagnostic bifocal lenses make lens fitting much easier and improve success. Lenses with a concentric annular design must center well. This ensures that some of the annular zone lies within the pupillary area, allowing the patient to perform near tasks (typing at a computer terminal, reading sheet music, and so on) while gazing in the primary position.

Aspheric variable focus lenses typically must be ordered 4 to 5 D steeper than comparable spherical lenses in order to achieve centration. If proper centration is not achieved, the patient will experience distance blur.

Translating, alternating image bifocal contact lenses come in two forms: segmented or concentric designs. These lenses must be fit such that the lens moves upward so the patient looks through the bifocal portion of the lens when reading. Conversely, when the patient is looking in the primary position of gaze, the bifocal must be below the pupil so as not to interfere with distance vision. Segmented design lenses must not rotate because the bifocal segment should be positioned just inferior to the pupil at all times. This is not a concern with concentric design lenses.

Monovision

Monovision, in which one eye is corrected for distance vision and the other eye is corrected for near, was first introduced by Westsmith more than 30 years ago (Fonda, 1966). The concept remains as controversial now as it was then. At best, monovision represents a compromise. The "side effects" of this treatment modality are well known: reduced vision in one eye, reduced binocularity, and diminished night vision. Many patients, however, quickly adapt to these problems (Erickson, 1988; Leboe and Goldberg, 1975; McGill and Erickson, 1988; Schor et al., 1989).

Ocular disorders that typically accompany old age may actually make prescribing monovision lenses easier. For example, the older patient may have anisometropia secondary to lens-induced myopia or implantation of an intraocular lens. Many of these patients have already adapted to the visual changes associated with their naturally occurring anisometropia. Obviously, the more myopic eye can be fit with a lower power contact lens, making reading possible.

Contact Lens and Glasses Combination

For some older patients the best solution is simply prescribing contact lenses for distance and spectacles for near. This technique works well with individuals who want to wear their contact lenses intermittently. For those patients who have difficulty adapting to the full add power of the bifocal contact lens, you can also prescribe a lower power bifocal contact lens augmented with reading glasses when needed.

CHALLENGES
Difficulties in Handling Lenses

Physical or medical problems make contact lens insertion, removal, and cleaning difficult for many older patients. Years of physical labor toughens hands with callouses, diabetic peripheral neuropathy reduces sensation to fingers and hands, parkinsonism results in tremors, and arthritis may gnarl and cripple fingers. Fortunately, these limitations do not necessarily have to prevent patients from wearing contact lenses.

First, be prepared to devote time to training. Older adults have a great capacity to learn but usually take a little longer to master something new. For the older contact lens patient, practice makes perfect. The contact lens assistant must patiently demonstrate and teach insertion and removal techniques and lens care. A rubber suction cup may make contact lens removal easier for some patients. When necessary, a family member can be taught how to insert and remove the contact lenses.

Dry Eyes

The precorneal tear layer performs many important functions. Tears wet the eye and contact lens to produce a smooth optical surface, flush the eye and contact lens of debris, maintain soft lens hydration, and fight infection. Unfortunately, as many as one third of patients over the age of 40 have clinically significant dry eyes (White and Gilman, 1991).

Obviously, it is important to evaluate the patient's tear layer carefully. The tear prism (lacrimal meniscus) along the lower lid margin should extend approximately 1 mm out onto the lid and have about a 1 mm height along the cornea. A decrease in the lacrimal lake occurs with a reduction in the aqueous layer of the tear film. This layer is important because it contains proteins and inorganic salts, substances that can coat a contact lens and produce deposits. The aqueous layer also includes lysozyme, an important antibacterial agent. Decreased TBUT and excessive debris also should be noted. A TBUT of less than 10 seconds is considered abnormal, indicative of a mucin layer deficiency.

A moderately dry eye does not automatically rule out contact lenses. First, the practitioner must determine the normal state of the tear film, conjunctiva, and cornea for the patient. Several ophthalmic dyes such as sodium fluorescein, rose bengal, alcian blue, and trypan blue can be used to determine the extent of drying of the cornea and conjuctiva. Fluorescein staining indicates disturbed epithelial cells. Rose bengal stains devitalized cells. Abnormal mucus is stained by alcian blue, while trypan blue stains mucous and dead cells. Drawings and photographs of the staining can be used to determine a baseline from which to monitor contact lens-induced changes.

Older patients with moderately disturbed tear layers can successfully wear contact lenses if various contact lens lubricants and wetting agents are used. Drops containing hydroxypropyl-methycellulose, polyvinyl alcohol, hydroxyethyl-cellulose, and sodium chloride replenish the tear layer and help wet and lubricate the contact lens.

Eyelid and Conjunctival Disorders

Inspect the lids for apposition abnormalities. Significant ectropion, entropion, trichiasis, and blepharochalasis should be corrected surgically before contact lens wear.

Carefully examine the patient's eyelids and lashes. Inspect the lid margins for inflammation, crusting, collarettes, chalazia, and hordeola. Also note inspissation of the meibomian glands. Treat the blepharitis and meibomianitis with lid soaks and scrubs, gland expression, and antibiotics. Acute chalazion and hordeolum should be treated with warm moist soaks and topical antibiotics. If conservative treatment fails, consider steroid injection of the chalazion or incision and curettage.

Evaluate the bulbar conjunctiva for xerosis, Bitot's spot, pinguecula, pterygium, or other changes associated with chronic dry eye or irritation. Use drawings and photographs to document these pre-contact lens abnormalities and attempt to clear up or minimize those problems that are treatable. Pinguecula and pterygium may lead to 3 and 9 o'clock staining with contact lens wear. Contact lenses are contraindicated in patients with an active pterygium.

Many older patients with glaucoma undergo filtering procedures to decrease intraocular pressure. Patients are often left with large cystic conjunctival blebs. The practitioner should approach the contact lens fitting of these patients with great caution. Contact lenses may irritate or conceivably rupture the bleb, leading to infection and endophthalmitis. Whether contact lenses should be used for patients with filtering blebs is a matter of clinical debate. The general consensus is to refrain from lens use for eyes with blebs if acceptable alternative optical corrections are tolerated. If contact lenses are prescribed for patients with large, overhanging cystic blebs, use small gas-permeable lenses that do not compromise the bleb. Patients who have flattened or shallow blebs with smooth borders may be fit with rigid lenses or hydrogels. The authors have limited their prescription of contact lenses in patients with filtering blebs to cases with irregular astigmatism or unilateral aphakia. The patient, however, must be fully informed concerning the possibility of infection.

SUMMARY

As "baby boomers" reach their golden years, they represent a tremendous opportunity for the contact lens practitioner. The doctor must abandon stereotypical attitudes concerning the aging patient. Older individuals have many unique visual needs and requirements that may be best met with contact lenses.

Primary consideration must be given to ocular health and integrity when considering contact lens applications for older patients. Systemic factors must also be taken into account. Dry eyes will be a major obstacle to overcome if these patients are to wear contact lenses successfully. The patient's personal needs and motivation must also be taken into account. Many patients will be happy with intermittent wear schedules.

REFERENCES

Andres S, Henriques A, et al. Factors of the precorneal fluid break time (BUT) and tolerance of contact lenses. Int Contact Lens Clin 1987;14:81–120.

Bennett E S. Basic fitting. *In* Bennett ES, Weissman BA (eds). Clinical Contact Lens Practice. Philadelphia; J.B. Lippincott, 1991, pp 1–22.

Caplan L, Molinari J. Clinical investigation of the Salvatori Sof-Form bifocal. Int Contact Lens Clin 1984;11(3):157–160.

Dart JK. Predisposing factors in microbial keratitis: The significance of contact lens wear. Br J Ophthalmol 1988;72:926–930.

Erickson P. The potential range of clear vision in monovision. J Am Optom Assoc 1988;59:203–205.

Fonda G. Presbyopia corrected with single vision spectacles or contact lenses: Preferences to bifocal contact lenses. Trans Ophthalmol Soc Aust 1966;25:46–50.

Hamano T, Mitsunaga S, Kotani S, et al. Tear volume in relation to contact lens wear and age. CLAO J 1990;16:57–61.

Leboe KA, Goldberg JB. Characteristics of binocular vision found for presbyopic patients wearing single vision contact lenses. J Am Optom Assoc 1975;46:1116–1123.

Liotet S, Guillaumin D, Cochet P et al. The genesis of organic deposits on soft contact lenses. CLAO J 1983;9:49–56.

MacKeen DL. Testing the tears. Contact Lens Spectrum 1986;1:36–38.

McGill E, Erickson P. Stereopsis in presbyopes wearing monovision and simultaneous vision bifocal contact lenses. Am J Optom Physiol Opt 1988;65:612–626.

Omerod LD. Causes and management of bacterial keratitis in the elderly. Can J Ophthalmol 1989;24:112–116.

Schor C, Carson M, Peterson G, et al. Effects of interocular blur suppression ability on monovision tasks performance. J Am Optom Assoc 1989;60:188–192.

Smedley TC, Friedrichsen SW, Cho MH. A comparison of self assessed satisfaction among wearers of dentures, hearing aids, and eye glasses. J Prosthet Dent 1989;62:654–61.

Stewart CR. Blinking and corneal lens wear. J Am Optom Assoc 1971;42:262–264.

Tripathi RC, Tripathi BJ, Rubin M. The pathology of soft contact lens spoilage. Ophthalmology 1980;87:365–380.

Tripathi RC, Tripathi BJ. The role of the lids in soft lens spoilage. CLAO J 1981;7:234–240.

US Department of Health, Education and Welfare. Refraction status and motility defects of persons 4–74 years. Vital Health Statistics: Data From the National Health Survey, US Public Health Service, 1971–72, pp 1–29.

White P, Gilman E. Preliminary evaluation. In Bennett ES, Weissman BA (eds): Clinical Contact Lens Practice. Philadelphia; J.B. Lippincott, 1991, pp 1–18.

9

Assessment and Management of Older Persons with Hearing Impairments

Rachel Negris
Sheree J. Aston

The National Center for Health Statistics estimates that there are 21 million Americans with hearing impairments; however, the incidence of hearing loss in the United States increases from 20% to almost 50% in those over 65 years old (Wax and DiPietro, 1984; Cox and McFarland, 1982). Furthermore, statistics show that age-related hearing loss is more common and more severe in males (Cox and McFarland, 1982).

Eyecare for this special population is both unique and necessary because

- Communication difficulties may create a barrier for an individual seeking eye care.
- As hearing decreases, sight becomes increasingly important.
- Among the population with hearing impairment there is a substantially greater incidence of ocular anomalies (refractive, binocular, and pathologic).

Older people with hearing impairments are a unique population for the eye care provider. One can imagine the difficulties a hearing-impaired person encounters in the course of an optometric examination. Consider the dim lighting and the visual barriers created by the equipment placed between the doctor and patient. Overall, decline in hearing acuity increases the isolation, vulnerability, and frustration often experienced by an elderly person.

DEFINITION OF HEARING IMPAIRMENT

There are four types of hearing losses defined by the dysfunctional area of the auditory pathway: conductive, sensorineural, mixed, and central.

Conductive hearing losses are created by disease or obstruction to the outer or middle ear. With conductive hearing loss, all frequencies of sound are usually evenly affected, and impairment is usually not severe (DiPietro, 1987). Hearing aids are often useful, and medical or surgical remediation is often possible. Sensorineural hearing loss involves the cochlea (sensory) or auditory nerve (neural). Hearing impairment is variable from mild to profound, and some sound frequencies (especially high frequencies) are affected more than others. A hearing aid generally amplifies all sounds equally, so the sound may be distorted and useless (DiPietro, 1987). A mixed type of hearing loss results from dysfunction of the outer or middle and inner ear (DiPietro, 1987). A central hearing loss results from impairment along the auditory pathway through the brainstem to the auditory cortex (DiPietro, 1987).

AGE-RELATED HEARING LOSS

Presbycusis, age-related hearing loss, varies in severity and in prognosis for aural rehabilitation. Presbycusis is usually a sensorineural hearing impairment that may be accompanied by a central auditory loss. Auditory sensitivity and discrimination of speech are reduced, and high frequency tones are affected disproportionately. Loss for extremely high frequencies begins in childhood (10–19-years old) and progresses throughout life. Between the fourth and sixth decades the high frequency loss may produce a minimal impairment. In the seventh and eighth decade high frequency loss progresses, reducing speech discrimination (Cox and McFarland, 1982).

Since high frequencies are affected to a much greater degree than lower ones, speech intelligibility is distorted regardless of the speaker's volume. This becomes greatly pronounced in environments with background noise. Even mild sensorineural losses may show poor word recognition ability (Cox and McFarland, 1982).

THE EVALUATION

The audiologist identifies the type and extent of hearing loss as well as the ability to understand speech under a variety of conditions. An aural rehabilitation program is designed for the individual. Audiologic evaluation includes testing to determine the listener's ability to receive and understand speech (Cox and McFarland, 1982).

The two primary tests are pure tone (sounds of a single frequency) and speech. Frequency is measured from 250 to 8000 Hz. The most important frequencies for speech are 500 to 3000 Hz. The loudness level required to hear a particular frequency is measured in decibels (dB). Normally, conversational speech is in the 40 to 50 dB range. The degree of hearing loss is described by responses to tones at increasing decibel levels (Cox and McFarland, 1982).

Speech discrimination testing measures the ability to understand speech if it is made sufficiently loud. Because some frequencies are affected more than others, sometimes even at maximum volume, elements of speech are missing and therefore distorted (Cox and McFarland, 1982).

MANAGEMENT
Coping

Hearing-impaired older adults are coping with a great disadvantage in society. They have different strategies for dealing with missing auditory input. Some people with recent-onset hearing loss may maintain that "nothing has happened." In conversation they may pretend to understand and nod in agreement. This form of denial does not help one cope effectively and is not likely to conceal the problems from others (Wax and DiPietro, 1984; Higgins, 1980).

Another compensation tactic is alertness—using situational cues for missed auditory information. Increasing visual alertness may be an effective strategy in some situations. Another strategy may involve a hearing companion. The hearing person finds out the needs of the hearing-impaired person to avoid communication difficulties and embarrassment. This may create stress within a family by increasing dependency and control.

A healthy coping strategy involves the open acknowledgment of the disability. In this way a person can manage a situation to improve interaction and communication. The person may suggest changes in seating, lighting, or reduction of background noise to facilitate communication (Wax and DiPietro, 1984; Higgins, 1980).

The concept of self is challenged throughout life by changes involved in maturation. Wax and DiPietro (1984) describe some of the defense mechanisms used to preserve one's identity in the face of hearing loss. One is avoidance of reality by denying a loss exists or blaming the environment or the speaker for lack of comprehension. Some individuals may acknowledge the reality of disability but use socially acceptable explanations for lack of understanding. They may devalue a desired experience. Instead of admitting that a hearing loss created difficulty at a movie, the hearing-impaired person may say that a movie was disappointing. Another strategy is rationalization, or making an undesirable situation look better. They may say that having a loss of hearing means "no more distractions" and they have "more peace and quiet" (Wax and DiPietro, 1984).

Remediation of Hearing Loss

In addition to an audiologic evaluation, a medical evaluation by an ear, nose, and throat physician is recommended. Presbycusis and noise-induced hearing loss is generally medically untreatable, but other causes of reduced hearing should be ruled out. A conductive hearing loss, such as otosclerosis, affects the bones of the middle ear. A hearing aid is often useful. In severe hearing impairment due to otosclerosis, surgical correction is sometimes possible. The affected ossicle may be removed and replaced with a prosthesis. Another potentially treatable conductive hearing loss is otitis media. This acute or chronic infection of the middle ear is most common in children and can be treated medically. Left untreated, otitis media can lead to severe permanent hearing impairment.

When the hearing impairment is determined to be sensorineural, differentiation of sensory (cochlear) versus neural (eighth cranial nerve) and central hearing loss is clinically important. Sensory losses may be caused by the use of systemic drugs that are ototoxic, by acoustic trauma or other local abnormality, or by neural causes (which are potentially life threatening). Cerebral vascular accident, mass lesion, or trauma can create central hearing loss. In the majority of cases, sensorineural hearing loss remains medically untreatable.

A cochlear implant is a medical device that bypasses the middle and inner ear. The auditory nerve is directly stimulated. Normal hearing is not imitated, but auditory information of tone and speech rhythms are used to improve speech reading and speech (Schleper, 1987).

After a complete evaluation a hearing aid may be prescribed. There are a variety of hearing aids available that are specific to the person's hearing loss and needs. Generally, a trial period with a new aid is recommended. An elderly person may be only partially assisted by a hearing aid due to problems of speech recognition, but a hearing aid may prove to be useful. Training sessions with the audiologist will be necessary to instruct the patient in the use of the aid.

Special Devices

In addition to personal hearing aids, there are many other assistive listening systems and signaling devices that may help the older person with hearing impairment. An audio induction loop provides amplification through the speaker's microphone and public address system along a wire that loops the seating area. The magnetic field is picked up by a hearing aid's telephone switch (DiPietro et al., 1984; Cox and McFarland, 1982). An audio loop can be used at home, wired to a television or radio. The wire loop surrounds the seating area. The volume on the hearing aid may be adjusted without increasing the volume of the television.

In the examination room, the doctor can use a wireless AM or FM system that transmits sound on radio wave to enhance communication with a hearing-impaired patient. These systems are used with and without hearing aids. Infrared systems are light-based systems used to direct speech to the hearing-impaired listener. They are used in conjunction with a receiver coupled to the hearing aid or to special receivers (DiPietro et al., 1984; Cox and McFarland, 1982).

Telephone use can be an obstacle to most hearing-impaired persons. Their telephones should be adapted to provide additional amplification in the hand set or by means of a portable amplifier. A telephone switch (T-switch) on the hearing aid enhances telephone use. A deaf person who cannot use a traditional telephone even with amplification may use a telecommunication device for the deaf (TDD). The phone handset is placed on the small Teletype receiver. Newer models do not require an external telephone; they may be connected directly to the telephone lines). The conversation is typed on a small keyboard. Signals are sent over the phone lines to be received by another TDD and read on paper or a display area. Some TDDs are computer-compatible and allow conversation between TDD and computer users with a modem. If the doctor's office does not have a TDD, a relay service is a reasonable alternative to transmission of messages through a family member or friend.

Alerting and signaling devices allow a hearing-impaired person to be aware of auditory signals (bells, alarms, buzzers). The signal may be visual (flashing lights), vibrotactile, or auditory (with an increase in volume). A flashing light may be used to signal the phone. The lighting system is sometimes used to signal different sounds. A wrist-worn vibrator is similarly used. Sound-sensitive transmitters are used to detect various sound sources and the wrist receiver vibrates; different lights on the receiver signal the source of the sound.

Access to television and films has been enhanced by means of closed captioning. A large portion of television programming is now closed-captioned. The hearing-impaired person uses a decoder built into or attached to a television set. The normally invisible information is decoded to a visible printed caption on the screen (DiPietro et al., 1984).

OPTOMETRIC EXAMINATION

The optometric examination of a person with hearing impairment is critically important. The incidence of visual disturbances is greater in the hearing-impaired population, and sight is relied upon for all interaction.

Communication

The mode of communication with the hearing-impaired will vary from person to person, and it is important to determine the patient's preferred method. The communication may be auditory, with or without amplification. A combination of speech and/or speech reading is used by most hearing-impaired individuals to some extent. Sign language is used by many. Written communication may be preferred in medical interactions (Kaplan, 1989).

In the patient with presbycusis, external amplification may be helpful with or without a hearing aid. Assistive listening devices such as wireless AM or FM systems are useful investments for the practitioner caring for geriatric patients.

The patient may rely upon speech reading to some extent, but it should never be assumed that a person can "lip read" all speech. Words that appear identical on the lips are homophonic. Look in the mirror and silently mouth the following words: "maybe," "baby," and "pay me." Many words are completely hidden with little or no movement of the lips. Watch the words "call," "hear," or "look." Important information should be supplemented by writing. Speech reading is a learned skill that some people are more able to rely upon than others. The degree of hearing loss and the onset of hearing impairment will influence a person's ability to speechread and speak.

A form of manual communication may be the preferred mode of communication. Sign language has many forms and is not international (nor is it based upon the spoken language of any country). In the United States the most common conversational sign language is American Sign Language (ASL). ASL is a visually based language. It is not the simple substitution of a sign for a spoken word or writing in the air. It is not simply mime or gestures. Direct communication between doctor and patient by signing is ideal.

If the use of a sign language interpreter is necessary, they can be located through the Registry of Interpreters for the Deaf, which trains and certifies them. A code of ethics ensures confidentiality of encounters. An oral interpreter compensates for factors that make speech reading difficult: distance from the speaker, lighting, clarity of speech, and other barriers to a clear view of the speaker's mouth. A deaf adult who uses oral communication may use an oral interpreter in critical situations, such as in a courtroom, to ensure accuracy of understanding. This type of interpreter silently mouths the words of the speaker. It is unlikely that an oral interpreter will be used formally in a medical situation; however, if communication with the doctor is difficult, an informal interpreter may be used, such as a family member or friend whom the patient is able to speech read with greater ease.

Language skills vary greatly among deaf people. In the prelingually deaf population, fluency in English is variable. As with spoken English, some will read and write English fluently, whereas others, although not fluent, will use written English to communicate their needs. Some patients may prefer to use written language instead of a sign language interpreter for privacy in some interactions (Kaplan, 1989).

Preparation for the Examination

If a patient is identified as hearing-impaired, the preferred mode of communication should be determined prior to the examination. If sign language is the patient's preferred language and the doctor is not fluent, an interpreter will be necessary (Appendix 9-1). If telephone contact is necessary, and the patient uses a TDD, call the patient directly through a TDD or TDD relay service. The National Information Center on Deafness or The National Association of the Deaf may be of assistance in identifying a local TDD relay service (see Appendix 9-1). The office staff should be aware of the hearing impairment and the appropriate means of communication, including the use of a TDD or TDD relay. Assistants need to know the appropriate examination and communication modifications.

Examination Modification

Several aspects of the typical examination must be modified, and in some cases, additional testing will be indicated. A questionnaire is a useful tool in gathering the medical history. Make sure that terminology is clear and go over the questionnaire with the patient after completion.

Consider equipment that may create a barrier to visual communication. The phoropter should be avoided; the conversation involved in a subjective refraction will be invisible. Utilization of a trial frame, especially for the subjective refraction, will enhance communication and subjective responses. Some equipment will block communication but cannot be avoided. The patient must understand the testing procedures prior to the start of the test because it may not be possible to coach him or her during the test. For example, if the patient understands the purpose of tonometry or automated perimetry, and the necessary response or position, a positive outcome is more likely. Many actions in the course of a normal examination will also effectively block communication. Asking the patient to close the eyes or removing glasses of a hearing aid user whose aid is in the glasses will create a dual barrier to hearing and vision. Such things as turning away while speaking or turning off the lights, as well as the temporary bleaching out of vision after ophthalmoscopy (especially binocular indirect ophthalmoscopy) create barriers to communication with a hearing-impaired person. Table 9-1 provides tips for communicating with the hearing-impaired person.

In assumed presbycusis a referral to an audiologist and/or ear, nose, and throat physician may be pertinent if the patient has not pursued these services. The cause of hearing loss will be determined and the possibility of aural remediation will be explored. Social and psychological impact of hearing loss should also be considered. Various agencies and support groups are available to help the person cope with the daily difficulties and impact of hearing loss (see Appendix 9-1).

Table 9-1 Communicating with a Hearing-Impaired Person

- Face the patient at a distance of 3 to 6 ft when speaking. Do not turn away or cover your mouth when speaking.

- Do not shout or exaggerate mouth movements (overarticulate) when speaking.

- Speak at a normal pace, not too rapidly nor too slowly.

- Do not speak directly into the patient's ear. It will prevent the use of visual information on the face, and as loudness increases at a close distance, distortion of sound may also increase.

- Consider the background noise, music, or sound filtering into the examination room. This can create an extremely difficult listening environment.

- Lighting is important. Do not dim the lights excessively and avoid having lights shining behind the examiner, creating shadows or shining into the patient's eyes.

- Include the patient in all discussions.

- If the patient prefers to communicate with sign language and an interpreter is used, speak directly to the patient and the interpreter will facilitate the conversation. Do not speak directly to the interpreter.

- If the patient does not understand, rephrase the question or statement.

- Ask leading questions periodically to assess understanding. Do not mistake nodding for understanding.

Dispensing and Follow-Up Considerations

In prescribing standard spectacles, contact lenses, or low-vision aids, consider the intermediate distance viewing area critical. Visual communication is used to some extent by most hearing-impaired persons, whether to augment or replace auditory input in communication. Speechreading or sign language is most likely to occur at a distance of 3 to 8 ft. Progressive addition lenses have been particularly useful for persons with hearing impairment because they allow a range of clear intermediate vision necessary for communication. When changing to this modality, the optometrist should schedule a training session in the use of progressive lenses and a follow-up visit to discuss any difficulties encountered. The use of a hearing aid will require some adjustment of frames, and some hearing aids are incorporated into the temples.

The use of printed literature is quite useful. Printed handouts are available explaining most diagnoses including refractive errors, binocular anomalies, and pathlogy. Most patients do not remember everything that was said concerning a particular diagnosis, and communication barriers make it possible that the entire discussion was not understood. Instructional materials regarding contact lens care and handling is necessary to ensure success. Above all, treat hearing-impaired older adults with respect. Do not speak about them to a third person in their presence. Include them in all discussions regarding any findings and recommendations.

Hearing-impaired older adults are greatly dependent upon vision. They often do not seek eye care due to the communication difficulties encountered in a typical examination; however, as hearing becomes less acute, sight becomes more and more critical for communication and interaction with the world. Examination modifications and specialized testing will be necessary to provide comprehensive appropriate care. Resources, groups, literature, and technology can assist the provider in meeting the needs of the elderly hearing-impaired person. The eye care provider who understands their visual needs and takes the time to communicate with these patients will provide a valuable and rewarding service.

REFERENCES

Cox BP, McFarland WH. Audiologic aspects of aging. We are all aging. Gallaudet Today. Washington, Gallaudet University Press, 1982.

DiPietro LJ. Deafness: A Fact Sheet. Washington, Gallaudet University Press, 1987.

DiPietro L, Williams P, Kaplan H. Alerting and Communication Devices for Hearing Impaired People: What's Available Now. Washington, Gallaudet University Press, 1984.

Higgins P. Outsiders in a Hearing World: A Sociology of Deafness. Beverly Hills, CA, Sage Publications, 1980.

Kaplan H. Communication Tips for Adults with Hearing Loss. Washington, Gallaudet University Press, 1989.

Schleper D. Communicating with Deaf People: An Introduction. National Information Center on Deafness. Washington, Gallaudet University Press, 1987.

Wax T, DiPietro LJ. Managing Hearing Loss in Later Life. Washington, Gallaudet University Press, 1984.

Resources for the Hearing Impaired

American Speech-Language-Hearing Association
10801 Rockville Pike
Rockville, MD 20852
(301) 897-5700 (V/TDD)

A professional organization that provides public information on communication disorders, including hearing impairment and the role of speech and hearing professionals. It will provide names of certified audiologists and local services.

Association of Late-Deafened Adults
P.O. Box 641763
Chicago, IL 60664-1763
(312) 604-4192 (Voice/TDD)

ALDA is a self-help, social, support, and advocacy group for adults deafened after having normal hearing (and after having developed speech and language). Local chapters are available.

National Information Center on Deafness
Gallaudet College
800 Florida Avenue NE
Washington, DC 20002-3695
(202) 651-5051 (V)
(202) 651-5052 (TDD)

NICD provides information on all areas of hearing impairment: education, vocation, communication, sign language programs, law, technology, barrier-free design, and other services for deaf and hard-of-hearing people. A list of diverse publications is available from NCID including *Communicating with Deaf People: An Introduction, You and Your Deaf Patients, Directory of National Organizations of and for Deaf and Hard of Hearing People.*

Registry of Interpreters for the Deaf, Inc.
8719 Colesville Road   Suite 310
Silver Spring, MD 20910
(301) 608-0050 (Voice/TDD)

RID trains and certifies sign language interpreters. It will provide information on local sources of interpreters.

Self Help for Hard-of-Hearing People, Inc.
7800 Wisconsin Avenue
Bethesda, MD 20814
(301) 657-2248 (V)
(301) 657-2249 (TDD)

Information on coping with hearing loss, assistive devices. Advocacy. State chapters are available.

10

Assessment and Management of Elderly with Cognitive Impairment

Sheree J. Aston

COGNITIVE IMPAIRMENT

Cognitive impairment is a problem frequently encountered in optometric practices with a large percentage of elderly patients. Management of these individuals can be both rewarding and challenging. Optometrists are in the position to identify dementia in their patients and refer them for full evaluation and treatment. Awareness of and screening for a cognitive impairment in the older patient is critical for two reasons: (1) the early and proper identification of diseases responsible for dementia is critical to their successful treatment, and (2) it allows the optometric practitioner to provide the best overall care with a higher rate of successful patient management (NIH, 1987).

Cognitive impairment, dementia, confusion states, and for many years, organic brain syndrome, have been loosely and globally used to describe a multitude of older adults with memory impairments or altered mental functions (Levy, 1986). It is no wonder that optometrists and other health care practitioners are "confused" about this subject.

Cognitive impairment in the older adult is often caused by disease, medication, grief, or anxiety. Among the elderly, the syndromes most commonly associated with cognitive impairment are delirium, depression, and dementia (Warshaw, 1986). They differ in terms of cause, onset of symptoms, clinical pattern, and treatability. Distinguishing between these three syndromes is a critical yet challenging assignment for any health care practitioner. The assessment and management of cognitive impairment is a complex activity requiring a team of health care providers and the assistance of family members (Warshaw, 1986).

Cognitive impairment is a growing health and social issue. Approximately 5% of noninstitutionalized individuals older than 65 years and 20% of those older than 75 years experience some degree of cognitive dysfunction. The occurrence of dementing diseases increases with age, with its highest rate in elderly individuals over 75 years of age (National Institutes of Health, 1987). After the age of 90, the chance of a person becoming demented is close to one in three. The numbers of elderly persons affected by dementia are dramatically high in long-term care facilities (Kane et al., 1989). According to the literature, 50% to 80% of the aged in nursing homes have some degree of cognitive impairment (Kane et al., 1989).

DELIRIUM

Delirium is also referred in the literature as acute confusional state (ACS), acute brain syndrome, and toxic psychosis. The characteristics include rapid development of symptoms, fluctuation of cognitive functions (especially at night), disturbed sleep patterns, impaired memory, problems with orientation, reduced awareness of immediate environment, attention disorders, and improvement of cognitive function after treatment of underlying condition (Warshaw, 1986; Kane et al., 1989).

The hallmark of ACS is a major change in mental status from a previously normal state of mind over a matter of hours or days (Warshaw, 1986). Disorders that cause delirium among the aged include tumors, cerebral vascular disease, systemic infection, head trauma, cardiovascular disease, metabolic disorders, severe trauma, sensory deprivation, temperature regulatory disorders, and exogenous substances (Liston, 1982).

Many secondary factors contribute to or exacerbate the development of delirium, including sensory impairments, memory loss, substance abuse, sleep deprivation, and occurrence of acute physical illness in combination with a fragile psychological status (Warshaw, 1986; Liston, 1982).

Confusion in a patient should signal the optometric practitioner to search for an underlying cause. An accurate and complete history must be collected from friends and family of the patient. ACS does not usually follow an insidious course. A detailed history is needed to gather information on previous alcohol or drug abuse, recent changes in over-the-counter or prescribed medications, paranoia, sensory losses, complaints of physical pains, or other medical problems. A mental status screening test must be administered to determine level of confusion (Appendix 10-1). Patients with suspected ACS should be referred for full mental status testing, physical examination, and laboratory studies (Kane et al., 1989).

Management of ACS includes identification and treatment of the underlying cause of delirium. Delirious patients must be placed in a setting where they cannot cause physical harm to themselves or others. They are often restrained or sedated while under treatment. Recovery of the cognitive functions may involve a period of weeks or even months. The individual's home, rather than a hospital setting, is preferred because it is a familiar environment (Warshaw, 1986).

DEPRESSION

Depression or pseudodementia is another frequent cause of cognitive impairment among the elderly. The elderly are at a higher risk of depression because of a combination of common losses—personal (death of friends and family), economic (retirement), and physical (age-related physiologic changes and chronic diseases). In the elderly, the clinical symptoms of depression are often atypical.

Unfortunately, it is often very difficult to diagnose depression accurately in the older person. Clinical depression and its associated disorders, therefore, often remain untreated among the elderly population. It is estimated that between 10% to 15% of the elderly have symptoms of clinical depression (Levy, 1986).

A depressed patient may experience sadness, dismay, and a sense of worthlessness. When these feelings are related to the occurrence of physical illness, clinical depression often will become a symptom of the disease. A depressed person may suffer from disturbances in appetite, sleep, and energy levels. Another result may be a change in cognitive status. Depression or pseudodementia is often characterized by withdrawal, apathy, confusion, and memory problems. Clinical depression can easily be misdiagnosed as senile dementia (Warshaw, 1986). Table 10-1 distinguishes between the cognitive symptoms of depression (pseudodementia) and a true dementia.

The accurate diagnosis of depression is critical for effective treatment. A clinically depressed elderly individual must be referred for appropriate psychother-

Table 10-1   Dementia Versus Depressive Pseudodementia: Comparison of Characteristics

Characteristics	Dementia	Depressive Pseudodementia
Onset can be dated with some precision	Unusual	Usual
Duration of symptoms before physicians consulted	Long	Short
Rapid progression of symptoms	Unusual	Usual
Patient's complaints of cognitive loss	Variable (minimized in later stages)	Emphasized
Patient's description of cognitive loss	Vague	Detailed
Family aware of dysfunction and severity	Variable (usual in later stages)	Usual
Loss of social skills	Late	Early
History of psychopathology	Uncommon	Common
Specific memory loss ("patchy" deficits)	Uncommon	Common
Attention and concentration	Often poor	Often good
Patient's emotional reaction to symptoms	Variable (unconcerned in later stages)	Great distress
Patient's efforts to cope with dysfunction	Maximal	Minimal

Adapted with permission from Small GW, Liston EH, Jarvik LF: Diagnosis and treatment of dementia in aged. West J Med 1981; 135:469–481.

apy, drug treatment, and social support. In addition, depressed patients often benefit from counseling specific to their economic, social, housing, or personal losses. Depression correctly identified in the elderly is very treatable. The "symptoms" of dementia will be reversed with successful management of clinical depression (Warshaw, 1986).

DEMENTIA

Dementia is also known as chronic confusional state. It is commonly incorrectly viewed as the same as Alzheimer's disease. Confusional states or senile dementias account for 80% to 90% of all confusional states (Warshaw, 1986).

The evaluation of dementia includes the following (NIH, 1987; Levy, 1986):

1. Complete history: current medical problems, medications, systemic history, current symptoms, and onset of and progression of symptoms
2. Physical examinations: blood pressure, hearing, vision, orientation, memory function, mental screening test, behavior, neurologic testing, and other cognitive testing
3. Diagnostic studies: complete blood work, radiographic studies, and other tests such as urinalysis, ECG, and EEG

Senile dementias are reversible (treatable) or irreversible (untreatable) (NIH, 1987). Differentiation between the two types of dementia is critical to the patient's overall care and functioning (Warshaw, 1986; Kane et al., 1989).

Reversible Dementias

Reversible dementias are caused by intoxications, psychiatric disorders, metabolic disorders, nutritional deficiencies, vascular problems, viral or bacterial infections, space occupying lesions, and normal pressure hydrocephalus (NIH, 1987).

The onset of dementia is usually gradual. Initially, the afflicted person will appear forgetful and restless, with a growing tendency to misplace objects and repeat words and actions. As the dementing condition worsens, more changes in the cognitive status take place. Patients may become disoriented, fail to recognize family members and friends, have major changes in sleeping patterns, or exhibit inappropriate antisocial behavior. They may undergo hallucinations, delusions, and symptoms of paranoia. In some cases, there may be changes in visual perception or motor systems. The decline may be slow or rapid and range from a few months to several years (NIH, 1987).

Irreversible Dementias

The second type of senile dementias are not currently treatable. It is estimated that 5% of the elderly suffer from these senile dementias, although approximately 22% of 80-year olds are affected (Gurland and Cross, 1982). The dementing diseases are characterized by memory loss (recent memory first), decreased ability to comprehend or make decisions, dulled affect, and ultimately, a major change in personality. Eventually, the person will experience problems with swallowing, walking, bladder control, bowel functions, and mobility (Kane et al., 1989).

Senile dementia of the Alzheimer type or primary degenerative dementia is responsible for 50% to 60% of the senile dementias of the 65 + age group. It is currently the fifth leading cause of death of this age group in the United States. Multi-infarct disease or "hardening of the arteries" is another common cause of irreversible dementia (10%–20%). In the classic cases, it is easy to distinguish between Alzheimer's and multi-infarct disease. Table 10-2 provides the different characteristics of Alzheimer's and multi-infarct disease sufferers. Other causes of dementia include Pick's disease, Parkinson's disease, Huntington's disease, and progressive supranuclear palsy and other neurologic disorders (Warshaw, 1986).

Treatment of the Demented Patient

Underlying conditions and diseases should be treated with prescription medicines. It is not uncommon for the cognitive functioning of demented patients to be further impaired by a variety of a physical disorders. The identification and

Table 10-2   Alzheimer's Versus Multi-Infarct Disease: Comparison of Characteristics

Characteristics	Senile Dementia	Multi-infarct Dementia
Demographic		
Sex	Women more commonly affected	Men more commonly affected
Age	Generally over age 75	Generally over age 60
History		
Time course of deficits	Gradually progressive	Stuttering or episodic with stepwise deterioration
History of hypertension	Less common	Common
History of stroke(s), transient ischemic attack(s), or other focal neurologic symptoms	Less common	Common
Examination		
Hypertension	Less common	Common
Focal neurologic signs	Uncommon	Common
Signs of atherosclerotic cardiovascular disease or peripheral vascular disease	Less common	Common
Emotional lability	Less common	More common

Reprinted with permission from Kane et al. Essentials of Clinical Geriatrics. New York, McGraw Hill, copyright © 1989.

aggressive management of these other disorders can improve mental capacities. Other underlying causes of cognitive dysfunction such as depression, visual, hearing deficits, and vitamin deficiencies should be managed. It is vital that demented patients have optimal sensory input. Periodic hearing and vision evaluations and remediation must be included in the overall management of these individuals (Warshaw, 1986; Levy, 1986).

A structured, familiar, quiet environment is important to maximize the cognitive functioning of the demented patient. Environmental modifications can minimize confusion, reduce agitation, and enhance overall functioning. Organized daily routines of meals, exercise periods, and medication regimen will help to maintain a sense of order. A simple, uncluttered environment is recommended. Any potential safety hazards such as pointed furniture or household poisons should be removed (Warshaw, 1986; Levy, 1986).

Support to caregivers is important, including education on the course and consequences of the dementing disease. Psychological counseling for family members for emotional support is recommended. Respite centers are available to provide the family with a rest from the daily physical and mental stress of patient care (Levy, 1986).

Whereas no medical treatments presently exist, two major rehabilitation strategies, sensory stimulation and activity stimulation, are used to enhance overall functioning of demented patients. Sensory stimulation consists of activities designed to stimulate all of the senses—vision, hearing, touch, smell, and taste. Activity stimulation is a program that utilizes purposeful physical exercise and mental gymnastics. Tasks are geared to the person's level of functioning. Both programs are conducted in a comfortable, familiar setting with a small number of friends and family (Levy, 1986).

OPTOMETRIC MANAGEMENT
The History

A comprehensive history is the key to any optometric evaluation. In the case of demented patients, information must be gathered from the family and the patient. A chronological account of the patient's cognitive and sensory problems is needed, including the onset and duration of symptoms. A comprehensive medical health history is necessary, including relevant diseases, traumas, psychological conditions, nutritional imbalances, substance abuse, and use of prescription and over-the-counter medications (NIH, 1987).

Patients who appear confused should be screened with a brief mental status test. A useful tool is the short portable mental status questionnaire (see Appendix 10-1). This screening device requires only 5 to 15 minutes to administer. It has a fairly high rate of both false-positives and false-negatives; however, any type of confusional state or dementia will not be diagnosed with a screening test alone. Both positive and negative results from these screening devices must be considered along with the history and individual case scenario. It is critical that all suspected "dementias" be referred quickly to the patient's family doctor or geriatric physician for full evaluation and treatment (NIH, 1987).

Communication with the Demented Patient

Revitalization is a collection of techniques developed to improve communication with the demented patient, and its key elements are useful in communicating with patients with true cognitive impairment. It has verbal and nonverbal components. The verbal component involves slow speech, repetition, simple words, and concrete language. The nonverbal elements include touch, eye contact, positioning, supportive atmosphere, and a positive attitude (University of Miami, 1987).

It is important for the practitioner and staff to speak slowly to the demented patient. The demented patient does not function well in hurried and time-pressured situations. During the examination, the practitioner must speak slowly and allow greater time for a response. The patient should not feel pressured; this will only cause agitation and decrease communication. To elicit needed information, restate questions to the demented person or rephrase the request. If possible, use the patient's own words or phrases. This will help the demented patient to grasp an idea that is retrievable. Simplicity is the principle to follow throughout the eye examination (University of Miami, 1987).

It is important not to use open-ended questions, answering them is too complicated a task for the confused patient. Questions requiring "yes" or "no" answers are easier for the demented person to understand and to reply. Practitioners should use the person's name with the name of an object (e.g., Harry, look at the chart). Do not use words such as him, her, or it. Talk about one item, task, or thing at a time and one step at a time. For example, when taking a distance acuity, do not say, "Read the line." Instead, give the instruction as a series of directions: "Harry, look through the glasses. Do you see the chart? Do you see the letters on the chart? Read the first letter. Read the second letter. Read the third letter." It is hard for a demented person to understand complex or abstract ideas. They cannot easily reason. Therefore, speak in simple terms about observable events. Keep in mind that it is easier to show a picture than to describe it (University of Miami, 1987).

These verbal suggestions can be reinforced by nonverbal support. Gestures should accompany words of instruction. Practitioners should point to the visual acuity chart as they ask the patient to look at it and read the individual letters. The use of touch will increase the likelihood of response to the request. It also communicates warmth and caring. In addition, touch will prepare the patient to receive more information. The doctor should try to speak softly just before the touch so as not to startle the patient. An example would be to gently touch the shoulder before pointing to the chart. Eye contact between the doctor and patient is meaningful because it will help to hold the patient's attention. It will also assist the doctor in judging how much of the question or request was understood. Be aware of the patient's best side in the case of a hearing impairment. Doctors should position themselves close to the patient at the same level to hold eye contact and speak clearly and directly toward the patient's good side. This position will also enable the practitioner to maintain the individual's attention (University of Miami, 1987).

The examination process will be more effective in a supportive atmosphere. Keep criticism to a minimum. Make an effort to understand the patient's answers, even though they may be garbled or incomplete. Praise all efforts to communicate. Maintain social conventions such as addressing elderly individuals as "Mr." or "Mrs." *At all cost*, avoid baby talk or speaking in the third person with the individual present. The practitioner must be positive and patient during the entire examination process (University of Miami, 1987).

Patient Care Tips

Assess and modify the office environment to reduce clutter and noise. Patients will respond better without distractions. Take care to reduce interruptions and stressful situations during the examination. Make sure to have a family member present during the examination to make the confused person feel more comfortable. Recommend adjustment of the home setting to family and friends to improve functioning. Educate the family on the proper use of light, color, and contrast in the home to improve overall visual functioning. The examination should be done in two sessions to reduce patient anxiety. Depending on the cognitive function, consider an ocular evaluation in the person's home to maximize responses. It is essential that vision is corrected to *optimal* level to improve sensory input. Hearing and vision are critical to maximize cognitive abilities (Bleimann, 1985; Levy, 1986).

Avoid the use of medications with central nervous system side effects such as tranquilizers. These drugs can cause further intellectual decline and increase the older person's level of confusion. Use friends and family to assist in the management plan to increase patient compliance (Warshaw, 1986).

Communicate with gestures, pictures, colors, and symbols rather than the written word. Use the revitalization techniques discussed earlier throughout the examination process to improve optometric evaluation and management results. Train the office staff on how to improve the communication with and care of the confused patient. (Levy, 1986; University of Miami, 1987; Warshaw, 1981).

Networking is even more important when dealing with the demented older adult. The optometrist is in a position to provide other needed services for the demented patient and his or her family. Distribute social service information regarding resources such as day care centers, home health aides, and respite centers. Consider interaction with the patient's other health providers to maximize overall care and function.

Optometric practitioners can serve their elderly patients through proper screening and referral for identification and treatment of "confusion," as well as by effectively managing the vision care of persons who are cognitively impaired.

REFERENCES

Bleimann R. Psychological and behavioral aspects of aging. *In* Bleimann R (ed): Workbook on Optometric Gerontology. St. Louis, American Optometric Association, 1985.

Gurland BJ, Cross PS. Epidemiology of psychopathology and old age: Some implications for clinical service. Psychiatr Clin North Am 1982; 5:11–28.

Kane RL, Ouslander JG, Abrass JB. Essentials of Clinical Geriatrics. New York, McGraw-Hill, 1989, pp 81–106.

Liston EH. Delirium in the aged. Psychiatr Clin North Am 1982; 5:49–66.

Levy LL. Cognitive treatment. *In* Davis LJ, Kurland M (eds): The Role of Occupational Therapy with the Elderly. Rockville, American Occupational Therapy Association, 1986, pp. 289–323.

National Institutes of Health Consensus Conference: Differential diagnosis of dementing diseases. JAMA 1987; 258:3411–3416.

University of Miami. Communicating with the Cognitive Impaired. Miami, Division of Biomedical Communications, School of Medicine, 1987.

Warshaw GA. Management of cognitive impairment in the elderly. New Dev Med Sept 1986; 1(2):40–53.

Short Portable Mental Status Questionnaire (SPMSQ)

Questions	Scoring
1. What is the date today (month/day/year)?	0–2 errors = intact
	3–4 errors = mild intellectual impairments
2. What day of the week is it?	
3. What is the name of this place?	5–7 errors = moderate intellectual impairment
4. What is your telephone number? (If no telephone, what is your street address?)	8–10 errors = severe intellectual impairment
5. How old are you?	Allow one more error if subject had no grade school education
6. When were you born (month/day/year)?	Allow one fewer error if subject has had education beyond high school
7. Who is the current president of the United States?	
8. Who was the president just before him?	
9. What was your mother's maiden name?	
10. Subtract 3 from 20 and keep subtracting 3 from each new number all the way down to zero.	

Adapted with permission from Folstein MF, Folstein S, McHuth PR: Mini-mental state: A practical method for grading the cognitive state of patients for the clinician. J Psychiatr Res 1975; 12:189–198.

Index

The abbreviations *t* and *f* stand for table and figure, respectively.